Low Carb,
High Fat
Food Revolution

Andreas Eenfeldt, MD

Low Carb, High Fat Food Revolution

Advice and Recipes to Improve Your Health and Reduce Your Weight

Translated by Viktoria Lindback

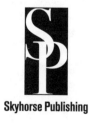

Skyhorse Publishing

TABLE OF CONTENTS

Two generations of Swedes have received incorrect dietary information . . . It is time to review the dietary guidelines and base them upon modern science.

GÖRAN BERGLUND
Professor of Internal Medicine, Lund University

INTRODUCTION

The revolution begins

He gave up and decided to eat himself to death. Sten Sture Skaldeman had failed in his last attempt at dieting and was more obese than ever. His heart could no longer effectively pump blood all the way around his large body. His blood pressure had skyrocketed. He could barely walk out to the mailbox. A doctor had given him six more months to live unless he lost weight.

Like many times before, he had tried eating less. Despite having tortured himself, the scale showed no progress. Nothing worked, so he gave up. During the remainder of his time alive, he planned on eating all of the food he had once tried to avoid. He was going to gorge on good food. The results were dumbfounding. A year later, he was thin and healthy.

The background

We thought we knew what healthy food was. Today, that world view is under attack. An increasing number of laymen, doctors, and professors ask the same question. Was it a mistake? Was it one of the most disastrous mistakes in the history of mankind?

It is 1958. The American scientist Ancel Keys is convinced that he has found the reason behind one of our deadliest conditions:

heart attacks. The cause, he thought, was fat. Eating fatty food increases the cholesterol in the blood, which in turn clogs the arteries in the same way fat clogs the pipes under your sink. His theory sounds about right, but the problem is, it lacks evidence.

It is 1984. As scientists continue to disagree, enthusiastic American politicians and lobbyists take matters into their own hands. It is time to teach everyone, the whole population, to eat less fat. New, "low-fat" products start to fill the grocery stores. They contain less fat but considerably more sugar and easily digested starch. It is an experiment of which no one can predict the results.

It is today. The world is heavier than ever, a victim of obesity and diabetes. An epidemic that started to accelerate in the 1980s. Perhaps you are one of the people with a couple of unwanted extra pounds? In the US, the home of low-fat products, the majority of the population has quickly become overweight or obese. That is three times more people than in the previous generation. People eat more calories than they expend. But why? It is time for us to realize that the answer is right in front of us.

The breaking point

What should you eat to stay or become healthy and thin? This question has never been more exciting, current, and controversial than it is today. Meanwhile, the confusion has never been greater. How do you know who to trust?

It took some time for me to figure it out. I went to medical school in the nineties and graduated in 2000, as scared of fat as any of my colleagues. Fat made you fat, they said. Saturated fat was definitely detrimental to the heart. I was happy to advise my patients and my own mother to avoid such dangerous food.

There was only one problem. Fewer and fewer people became healthier and thinner as the years went on. Most people slowly gained weight and required more and more medication for spiking blood pressure, blood sugar, cholesterol, aches, and so on. People grew heavier and sicker when they tried to live healthily.

Something wasn't right. I was not contributing to better health. I was perpetuating Western epidemics such as obesity, diabetes, heart disease, cancer, and dementia.

In retrospect, it was easy to see the issue with my medical education. It did not focus on health. It focused on diseases and the medications that cure, or more often reduce, disease symptoms. You have to learn about food and health elsewhere. I started to read more and more books, blogs, and hundreds of scientific research studies. Something was devastatingly wrong, and the reason became increasingly clear. Many had realized it much earlier and had written about it for decades.

Our ancestors did not suffer from today's endemic diseases. This has largely been explained by the fact that we have suddenly become gluttonous and lazy: we eat too much and run too little. But it turns out that this is far from the whole explanation. The old world view is eroding. We have made a huge mistake.

Modern science opens up a new way of approaching food and health. Healthier and thinner patients confirm that it works in reality as well. More and more doctors, laymen, and professors are reaching the same conclusions today. The new approach is spreading across the world and Sweden is pioneering the change. We have come the farthest and can pave the way.

Today, many people have stopped eating the industry's low-fat products, also known as fake food. That includes foods that are created in factories with the cheapest ingredients available: easily digested starch, sugar, plant oils, color agents, artificial flavoring, and additives. Fake food is recognized by its colorful packaging and nutrition labels that only chemists can explain. Advertising is trying to convince you that it is healthy, but you can easily see through it.

An increasing number of Swedes are stepping out in the media limelight to talk about how they have regained their health and lost weight. To everybody's surprise, they have done so by eating the opposite of what they had been previously recommended. We see these types of success stories every other day. But the weight loss is often not the most impressive part. It is obvious that it is not about dieting. It is about health.

Large scientific studies are starting to confirm what many people have already started noticing in their everyday lives. The pieces of the puzzle of the effect food has on health are starting to fall into place. The new view is becoming increasingly clearer—and it is surprising.

I had to help spread the new knowledge and contribute to change. In 2007, I started the Swedish blog kostdoktorn.se, which quickly became Sweden's largest health blog, with over ten thousand visitors per day. In 2011, I launched the English version, Dietdoctor.com. That is pretty indicative of the popularity of the subject. I can only agree. The story upon which this book is based is the most fantastic story I have ever heard. Hopefully you will agree.

Low Carb, High Fat Food Revolution is written for the modern reader who is ready to let go of outdated ideas, the kind of person who can tell the difference between credible science and the food industry's advertisements. You too can understand, try, and eat your way to better health and weight. Then you can help your loved ones do the same. It may sound silly, but it's true: if more people do the same, it might change the world.

The Revolution is here. With good conscience, you can eat yourself full again. Bon appétit!

I.

In retrospect

CHAPTER ONE

What are you designed to eat?

The dieting debate is hot in Sweden. What should you eat to become healthy and thin? Mediterranean food, the Paleolithic diet, or according to the Eatwell Plate model? Fat or carbohydrates, or maybe protein? Fibers or antioxidants? Fruit or no fruit?

There are a couple of high-profile experts that claim to know, but their theories differ from each other. Even relevant professors have completely different opinions. How do you know who to trust?

I say that there is a good way of finding out. Look at your body and study yourself: what are you designed to eat? You are the result of millions of years of evolution. Every cell in your body contains myriad genes, the refined blueprint of a human. Your genes are special. Your ancestors managed to pass them on to you. The same thing has taken place for millions of years, going back to your earliest ancestors on the African savannah. The same thing has taken place for hundreds of thousands of generations.

For every new generation, strong and beneficial genes had a better chance of making it into your family tree. Genes that provided strength and health during the conditions under which your ancestors lived. Genes that worked well with the diet that your ancestors ate.

In other words: your genes are designed for the food that your forefathers ate thousands of years ago. Today, we know some of what they ate and more importantly, what they *didn't* eat. With that knowledge in mind, you might be able to discern the mistake made by many dietary experts in the media.

You can compare it to a car. A car is designed by engineers to run on a certain type of fuel. It might be gasoline, diesel, or ethanol. If you fill up the car with the right fuel, the engine will run well. If you don't, it will run poorly, or not at all. In fact, they say that if you pour sugar into a gasoline tank, the engine will start to seize.

You are a lot more complex than a car. Your body is also designed to run on a certain type of fuel, namely, exactly what your ancestors ate. If you eat something else, your body will work poorly, or not at all.

In the Western world today, much of the dietary advice unfortunately prompts us to fill up with the wrong kind of fuel. Despite the good intentions, this has led to obesity and disease, which the scientific community has just started to investigate using large studies. More about that later. Modern science simply proves what should have been apparent a long time ago. What we knew, but accidently forgot.

The most remarkable fact is that a multitude of explorers and missionary doctors during the nineteenth and twentieth centuries started to tell the same story from all corners of the world. A story that, if true, could revolutionize our world as well as our health.

A mystery

Albert Schweitzer arrived in West Africa on April 16, 1913. He was a doctor and would later go on to receive the Nobel Peace Prize for his missionary work. On average, he met with thirty to forty patients per day. Most of them suffered from infections such as malaria. It took forty-one years before he saw an African patient with appendicitis. How is that possible? Appendicitis is a regular occurrence in modern emergency rooms.

It gets weirder. During his initial time there, Schweitzer didn't see one single case of cancer. Of course, he admitted later that there might have been some cases, but they were certainly rare.

However, during the latter part of his stay in West Africa, he treated an increasing number of cancer patients. Schweitzer suspected that this was caused by the fact that the local people had started living like their white visitors.

The Schweitzer story is just one among many. Cancer and appendicitis are just the beginning. Today's Western endemic diseases first appeared when Western food started to spread across the globe.

It is possible that we have ignored or misinterpreted what these stories mean. But let's return to the food, or the fuel, for which your body is designed. Let's return to a time in history prior to Albert Schweitzer's missionary work in West Africa. Let's rewind five million years.

Five million years worth of fuel

Our closest living relatives in the animal kingdom are chimpanzees, the smartest of the human apes. We are distant cousins, very distant. To make a family tree of our shared ancestors, we need to rewind five million years. Let's track evolution from there, up until today.

As you know, our forefathers, the humans-to-be, resided in Africa. A million years later, these ape-like creatures started walking around the savannah on two legs. That was only the beginning. Slowly but surely, during hundreds of thousands of years, our ancestors underwent tremendous transformation. Their brains became larger, they discovered fire and tools, and they developed a more advanced form of oral communication. They became humans. They became you and me. But what did they eat?

As you know, the African savannah did not have McDonald's four million years ago. Nor did it exist there when modern-day humans spread out throughout Africa some seventy thousand years ago. McDonald's didn't even exist in North America fifteen thousand years ago, when humans relocated from Siberia to Alaska and rapidly started to populate the New World.

McDonald's didn't exist anywhere at that point. Neither did soda, nor French fries. There also wasn't any bread, pasta, or potatoes. All of those things require agriculture, and we didn't develop those skills until later on. So what did we eat throughout our long evolution?

Before inventing agriculture, we were hunter-gatherers. That means we consumed food readily available in nature. We hunted animals and ate them. We caught fish and ate it. We consumed every edible thing in nature: eggs, nuts, roots, fruit, and other edible parts of plants.

Those are the types of foods to which your genes have adjusted throughout millions of years. That is the type of fuel for which your body is designed. The food was nutritious, full of vitamins and minerals. We received plenty of protein and energy from fat and moderate amounts of indigestible carbohydrates.[1]

Easily digestible carbohydrates were rare; our ancestors ate almost no sugar or pure starch. Not in five million years. But then the world rapidly changed, in three steps.

The last day of the year

The agricultural revolution changed everything. It started nine thousand years ago, in today's Iraq, which at the time was a lot greener. After that, agriculture spread across the world. It arrived in the Nordics some four thousand years ago.

Farming enabled us to grow our own food. We could extract a lot more food from the same amount of land than when we were hunter-gatherers. Population density increased, cities started to arise, and civilization picked up speed. Agriculture brought along a lot of positive change, but also a set of new problems. We will focus on one: what were the consequences for our health?

---

1. A leading expert, Professor Loren Cordain, estimates that hunter-gatherers consumed significantly less protein than we eat today, along with a reduced amount of carbohydrates (often significantly less) and more fat. The carbohydrates were more diluted and indigestible: roots, nuts, wild fruit, and parts of plants. No pure sugar or starch.

You can read more about the science in the reference section in the back of this book. If you are like me and find it interesting, there are references to a couple of hundred scientific studies. Either way, you will be fine. Humans, like all types of animals, are able to eat really healthy food without first analyzing and debating its molecular contents. There are easier ways of identifying real food.

The agricultural food was different from what we had eaten before: bread, rice, potatoes, pasta, and other farmed products that mostly consist of starch. Starch is long-chained glucose, which is broken down into pure glucose in your stomach. We will have good reason to return to the meaning of this later. The fact is, food for which your body is not designed could have unwanted effects on your health.

Thousands of years of agriculture sounds like a long time. But it is not a long time, compared to the vast amount of time it takes to fundamentally change our genes and the way our body works. For the purpose of this analysis, let's condense human evolution from the time we separated ourselves from our genetic relatives into one year. In other words, let's have a look at human evolution as if it was taking place during one year.

In this scenario, we were hunter-gatherers for about 364 days, until early on New Year's Eve. During the last day of the year, agriculture spread across the planet. That changed our food, and the question is whether or not we had ample time to acclimate in such a short time frame, or, in other words, whether or not that kind of food is perilous for our health.

Recently, we experienced the biggest transformation of the three, a transformation to which we have had very little time to adjust. In relation to the yearlong human evolution, this change came about approximately fifteen minutes before the stroke of midnight on New Year's Eve. Just in time for popping the champagne and celebrating the midnight toast. I am referring to the transformation of which Albert Schweitzer and others saw the effects.

The industrial revolution came with factories that produced new types of food. Agriculture had increased our intake of starch, which becomes pure glucose in our stomachs. The industrial revolution perpetuated this change. Factories found cheap ways to grind white flour, in which everything but the pure starch is removed. This had several economic advantages. The new white flour could be stored for long periods of time without attracting vermin due to the low nutritional value, since they cannot subsist on pure starch. That meant the flour could be shipped around the world as a trade commodity.

The industrial revolution gave us an additional commodity that could be shipped across the world. Something sweet that had, up until this point, been a luxury good and could now be produced cheaply and in large quantities in factories. This gave more people—almost everybody—the opportunity to eat and drink as much sugar as they wanted. In large quantities, sugar has even more detrimental health effects than starch.

Wherever sugar and starch could be found in the world, the same thing happened. The spread of Western food was followed by one or two decades of unexpected consequences.

The third and last transformation of our diet remains. It may have taken place during your lifetime, unless you are too young— it occurred just a couple of decades ago. In relation to the year-long human evolution, it took place during the New Year's Eve midnight countdown, as you are starting to raise your glass. The fear of fat and cholesterol exacerbated the changes that had taken place before. This fear resulted in many people eating more of the new food and a slowly emerging endemic disease. Today's ongoing disaster is the subject of chapter two.

However, before we get to that, part of the history lesson remains. We know a lot about the consequences of the first transformation, agriculture. We also know a lot about what took place during the industrial revolution, the second change. But what happens when you eat the new food, or in other words, easily digestible carbohydrates?

Five grams of sugar

When you eat bread baked with white flour, also known as pure starch, it quickly breaks down to pure glucose in your stomach. In turn, it is quickly absorbed into the bloodstream and raises the blood sugar. Your body is not designed to handle a lot of pure starch.

Do you know how much blood sugar your blood currently contains? Approximately five grams, or one teaspoon, of glucose. That's it, mixed with five liters of blood if you're healthy. But that can change.

Your blood sugar normally fluctuates between set limits. It never rises a lot after the intake of food. For healthy people, it rises no more than 50 percent. In fact, high blood sugar levels can actually harm the arteries.

How does the body handle large blood sugar spikes caused by starch? How does the body manage to still maintain a normal blood sugar level? The answer is that the blood sugar is absorbed and used by the cells. That process requires a signal from a hormone that plays a central role in our body and our history. It is called insulin.

Insulin is crucial for regulating the blood sugar that was developed during the period we did not consume starch. If you eat a big bowl of pasta, rice, or potatoes, over a hundred grams of glucose flood your bloodstream, when your blood is only supposed to contain five grams' worth. The result? The insulin skyrockets, potentially to abnormal levels, to attempt to stabilize the blood sugar.

The more starch you eat, the higher the insulin level.

Insulin is also the body's fat-storing hormone. For that and a plethora of other reasons, elevated insulin levels could be harmful. Among populations that didn't eat the new food, the insulin levels were a lot lower than what is normal today.

That was theory. How about a dose of reality from one of the most famous Swedes of all times; the man featured on the Swedish 100-crown bill?

Diet has a great effect on the inhabitants of a country. A Lapplander, or Saami [denomination of someone from the north of Sweden] lives on meat, fish, and birds, and is small, slim, light, nimble; but a farmer in the south of Sweden, in the plains of Skåne, who eats a lot of buckwheat porridge, and whose food consists chiefly ex vegetabilibus farinaceis [vegetable flour dishes], grows big, coarse, stout, strong, sluggish, heavy.

CARL LINNAEUS
From his book SKÅNSKA RESA, 1751

What the perceptive Linneaus observed in the eighteenth century was only a preview of what was to come. He had just seen the effects of the first transformation, agriculture (which existed in the south, but not in northern Sweden).[2]

The next big transformation of our food was on its way. Soon you wouldn't need his intellect to notice the difference.

The luxury of kings becomes everyday food

In the eighteenth century, Swedes ate around 0.22 lbs (0.1 kg) of pure sugar per year. In 1850, that amount had increased to 8.8 lbs (4 kg). Today, the number is 99 lbs (45 kg). In the US it is even worse. Pure sugar that was a rare luxury commodity during the Middle Ages has since become cheaper and more commonplace. We can attribute that to the Industrial Revolution and its factories.

The chart below shows the dramatic change of the consumption of pure sugar (in kilos per person and year) in the Western world since the eigteenth century.

Pounds of sugar per person per year

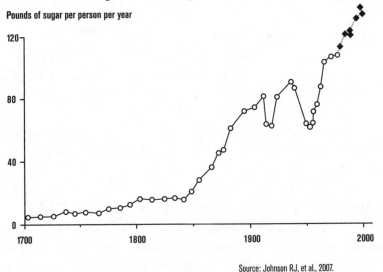

Source: Johnson RJ, et al., 2007.

---

2. Skåningarna [denomination for southern Swedes] could have been aware of the issue themselves. An old Swedish song starts: "You skåningar, you skåningar, tomorrow you will eat oatmeal, and dip it in honey so that you become thick and fat. . . ."

The numbers derive from England up until 1975, and thereafter from the US (represented by black squares on the curve). The two big dips occurred during the world wars when food was rationed. In a couple of hundred years, we have gone from almost no sugar to an abundance thereof. What does that mean? Is there a risk in eating tens of kilos of sugar?

The pure white sugar does not only contain glucose like starch. White sugar only consists of 50 percent glucose. The rest is fructose.

Throughout our evolution, we did not consume large quantities of fructose. We are not designed for it. In modern scientific studies, fructose (especially in large quantities) is the worst carbohydrate for your health and weight. But that type of science will have to wait.

One thing is clear: if you want to improve only one single thing in your diet, you should stop eating sugar.[3] There is probably nothing else that could improve your health more easily.

What happened when the food of the Industrial Revolution, pure sugar and white flour, spread across the world? We have many sources that can tell the story.

Indiana Jones as a dentist

No story is perhaps as good as that of Weston A. Price, an American dentist that during the 1920s and 1930s visited primitive populations around the world with his wife. He was obsessed with finding what obviously made them so much healthier. The couple visited Australian aborigines, Polynesians in the Pacific Ocean, Eskimos, South and North American Indians, isolated villages in the Swiss mountains, and African tribes.

They traveled to some of the most remote and isolated areas imaginable by airplane, river rafts, and hiking through jungles, and tried to communicate with natives using body language. I imagine Price's trips to be similar to those of Indiana Jones.

---

3. The quickest way of consuming enough sugar to become obese and ill is to drink soda or juice. Drink water instead. A glass of wine might even be better for your health.

He describes his trip and findings in the book *Nutrition and Physical Degeneration* from 1939. I have the seventh edition of this undeniable classic. Unfortunately, Price didn't have the same storytelling talent as Steven Spielberg. His rather dry account of his astounding findings is crammed with long tables showing the number of dental cavities he found. Price was primarily a dentist. After a suitable gift to the chieftain, the local populations seem to have been lining up to get their teeth examined and photographed.

The tables are clear. Those who didn't eat our modern food didn't have a single cavity. Those who ate a lot of it had plenty. The numbers don't lie. But it is not the numbers that are unforgettable, it's the photographs.

These primitive populations, photographed during the early twentieth century, did not have dentists. They didn't even have toothpaste or modern toothbrushes. Despite this, they stood there smiling with bright white teeth that would make anyone in Hollywood jealous. That was what it looked like regardless of where Price traveled, before sugar and white flour had appeared. The rest of the story is easy to predict.

For every primitive population that Weston A. Price visited, he also sought out the subset of them that lived close to the Western civilization: in the seaports where they ate Western food, and among people who worked on sugar plantations. These people still didn't have access to modern dentistry or good habits. When they ate sugar and white flour, it was apparent in their mouths.

The photos from the seaports were the complete opposite of the ones from the remote villages. The people had broken teeth. Terrible cavities. All of the issues you only see in Sweden today with people who don't take care of their teeth at all: addicts, mentally ill people, and a few who suffer from odontophobia.

Sugar and white flour make your teeth rot unless you can diligently brush them. Without sugar and starch, you do not get cavities, not even if you ignore brushing. Skeletons from the Stone Age show almost no cavities, even if the human lived to be sixty years old.

This wouldn't surprise a dentist. Caries-associated bacteria subsist on sugar, which it ferments to acid, which could corrode your teeth.

Despite the absence of dentists back then, their teeth were cavity-free when they ate the food for which our bodies are designed. If sugar and white flour can make your teeth rot, in what other ways can they harm the rest of your body?

So close to the truth

The sugar industry naturally doesn't admit to sugar being harmful. When it comes to our dental health, it is difficult to hide, even if they try to do so. For example, Danisco Sugar recently wrote on its website that dental cavities are not caused solely by sugar, but "primarily by poor and insufficient brushing." With the same logic, cyanide is probably nothing to worry about, since the danger is mostly the absence of an antidote.

Using different arguments, sugar producers try to avoid the obvious correlation with obesity, diabetes, and other Western diseases. Unfortunately, they have been successful, although we should have known better a long time ago.

The fact is, we were so close. So close to connecting all the dots. In the middle of the twentieth century, what doctors were reporting could have given us the answer. They reported the effects of the big change, the white flour and sugar. They reported how diseases had changed across the world. It was all compiled by someone who should have been revered, who should have received the Nobel Prize.

In the British Navy

Thomas Latimer Cleave was born in 1906. His sister died young from appendicitis. That is only one of the diseases for which he would come to propose a cause. After having trained to become a doctor, he was hired by the British Navy. His friends and colleagues called him "Peter."

He worked in the British Navy's hospital in Hong Kong and Malta, so he got to see how diseases manifested themselves among different populations. During World War II he worked as a doctor on a warship. Something started to dawn upon him. After the war, he wrote letters to hundreds of doctors around the world. He asked about the occurrence of specific diseases. The new diseases.

Cleve had been deeply influenced by Darwin's theory about evolution and natural selection. Every species progressively adapts to its environment, but it takes time. The risk with new environmental elements, such as food, is based on the time we have to adjust to it. Pure sugar was the newest addition and the consumption thereof had skyrocketed.

Cleave saw things that had existed in the human environment as natural. Food that is similar to humans' original diet is what I call "real food" in this book; the type of food that makes you healthy.

Cleave noted a long list of new diseases that had suddenly become prevalent around the world in a few decades. That could not be natural. He could only make one conclusion. Our bodies were not ill-designed, just improperly used. The diseases included obesity, diabetes, heart disease, gallstones, cavities, constipation, ulcers, and appendicitis.

He started publishing texts about his theory in 1955 and summarized his research in *The Saccharine Disease* in 1974. Sugar and the white flour were regarded as the cause behind all of the Western diseases.[4]

Cleave was convinced that the issue was the purification and concentration of carbohydrates. It tricks us into eating more and can result in obesity over time. You don't gain weight by being gluttonous or lazy. He noted how no wild animals become obese, regardless of the amounts of food they have access to. Not when

---

4. In Swedish, the title would translate to "The Sugar Disease," since the starch in flour is broken down into glucose. Cleave thought it was an appropriate simplification.

Just like the book by Weston A. Price, this book can be read online for free. Just search for these titles online. I truly recommend them for all history buffs.

they keep their natural diet. The same should go for humans, but the problems arose with the new food.

Our knowledge about the full effects of sugar and starch on the blood sugar and insulin is still incomplete. Cleave's conclusions were based on how diseases spread through food and evolution theory. He got pretty close to the truth, despite not having access to modern science.

Cleave was intelligent and had refined his theory for decades. But he was an outsider. He ended his career as head of the Navy's medical research, but the Navy was not part of the research culture of academia. Cleave was different. While others were researching details in a laboratory, he was focused on the big picture. It was clear that he was not going to be taken seriously. Despite this, a couple of influential doctors and scientists took him under their wings.

Sir Richard Doll, one of the doctors who proved that smoking causes lung cancer, wrote one of the forewords for early versions of Cleave's book. If just a small share of the theory turned out to be true, he wrote, it would still contribute more to science than any of the big research institutions in a generation.

The famous doctor Denis Burkitt wrote the foreword to *The Saccharine Disease*. He had long worked in Africa and seen with his own eyes the differences in the disease climate around the world. He knew that what Cleave was saying was true and contacted many doctors across the world who confirmed. Burkitt compared the revolutionizing potential of the ideas to the discovery of bacteria, x-rays, and antibiotics. At one point, things looked promising for Cleave's theory. It could have changed the world.

But it wasn't that simple. There was a competing theory, and it had already gained traction with a charismatic figurehead.

The disaster begins

Everywhere in the world, the same thing happened once the new food arrived. Perhaps the question "What are you designed to eat?" should be rephrased "What are you not designed to eat?" The answer, from human history, is sugar and white flour.

Why did everyone start to think the complete opposite during the latter part of the twentieth century? Why was fat all of a sudden blacklisted? How did we end up like this? How did the Western world end up becoming the victim of what, in retrospect, could have been the most detrimental medical mistake ever?

The story is reminiscent of both a thriller and a catastrophe movie. Let us begin.

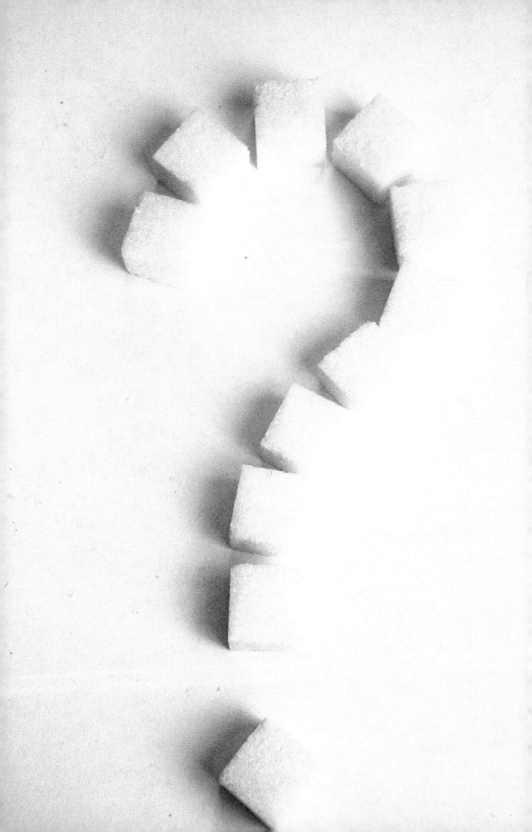

CHAPTER TWO

The mistake, the fear of fat, and the obesity epidemic

"Sorry, it's true. Cholesterol really is a killer. No fatty milk. No butter. No fatty meat . . . "

It is March 26, 1984, and the Americans were to be scared. They were to be scared of fat. The headline and the first sentences in a foreboding TIME magazine article leave no doubts. Neither does the cover, which featured a sad breakfast plate. The egg eyes and bacon mouth illustrate the sadness. The headlines say the rest: CHOLESTEROL—AND NOW THE BAD NEWS . . .

Today, with the beauty of retrospection and hundreds of millions of obese Americans later, it is worth looking back at this day in 1984.

Strangely enough, the media was reporting on a pharmaceutical research report. A cholesterol-lowering drug had been found to reduce the risk of having a heart attack. After a couple of failed attempts, it was the first study to put forth the theory about the danger of fat. It was a popular theory on which many politicians, scientists, and lobbyists had bet their careers. Finally they had their chance. But were they right?

If one pill results in fewer heart attacks for risk patients, does that prove that lean cuisine can make Americans healthier?

The answer is, of course, no. The fear mongering was a long shot. No one could know what would happen. The politicians and scientists who supported the theory were probably under the impression that they were doing some good and that the end justified the means. With their conviction that fat was dangerous, they relaxed the requirement for scientific proof. When we look back, the conclusion is evident. The emperor had no clothes that day. Conviction cannot replace proof.

In actuality, they were playing roulette with the health of the Western world, our health. They put everything on red. They took a massive risk. How did they end up there? We'll get to that later, but first, let's straighten something out.

How can it be dangerous to eat less fat? Aside from nutrient deficiency, how can *less* of something be dangerous?

You cannot eat significantly less of something without eating more of something else. Not if you want to feel full. If you eat less fat, you essentially have to eat more carbohydrates. That's because fat and carbohydrates are the main sources of energy in our diet. Protein and alcohol also give us energy, but only in small quantities.

If you eat less fat, you eat more carbohydrates. That is inevitable. Which carbohydrates? If you advise Americans to eat less fat, of what will they eat more? Just beans and sprouts? Or will they eat more . . . sugar and white flour? The new cheap food, that which causes blood sugar spikes and the fat-storing hormone insulin?

The food industry celebrated the new rules. From the EIGHT-IES and onward, it was able to produce food of the cheapest possible ingredients, sugar and starch, dilute it with water and additives, and sell it at a high price with the health-argument that it was "low fat." The boring taste could be disguised with added sugar, salt, and aromas.

Today we see the results of this lean cuisine experiment in the Western world's increasingly heavier populations. It is a scary picture. A complete epidemic of obesity and something called metabolic syndrome. Something we might as well rename the Western disease. And it comes with several of our new endemic diseases.

Good intentions

Let us rewind to 1958. They say the road to hell is paved with good intentions. The scientist Ancel Keys had the best of intentions. He wanted to rescue the Western world from its deadliest disease, and he thought he had found the answer. It was cholesterol. The cholesterol needed to disappear.

Keys was an only child born in 1904, and it would have been an understatement to call him driven. In his thirties he had already obtained two PhDs in biology and physiology.

Soon he led an expedition to the Andes to study how the body is affected by high elevation. He spent some time at an altitude of 20,000 FEET in the middle of the winter with night temperatures of around -49 degrees Fahrenheit (-45 degrees Celsius). A couple of participants became altitude sick (one almost died), but Keys managed well.

During WWII, he designed the army's rations, the so-called K-rations, with a K for Keys. One of those would give a soldier a daily dose of 3,000 calories, including chocolate, gum, and twelve daily cigarettes.

At the end of the war, Keys had just completed one of the most spectacular studies of his time, focusing on starvation. Today, this would hardly have passed ethical approval. He made thirty-six conscientious objectors participate in order to avoid the war. Instead they were starved and meticulously monitored for six months. On average, they lost 25 percent of their body weight.[5] But Ancel Keys became famous for something else later on. It was what would place him on the front page of *TIME* magazine and gave him the nickname "Mr. Cholesterol."

---

5. The starvations caused depression and anxiety for many of the participants. Some experienced reduced ability to concentrate and difficulty thinking clearly. Other reported side effects were obsession with thoughts of food, a significantly reduced sex drive, and social withdrawal. One participant cut off three fingers, perhaps to be dismissed from the study. In terms of changes to their bodies, they noted reduced metabolism and lower body temperatures and pulse. Many of the side effects that arose are common for eating disorders, such as anorexia and bulimia.

The starvation diet consisted of 1,560 calories daily of primarily starch, such as bread and potatoes. They were also forced to work hard and take walks. It is striking how similar this is to today's conventional weight loss advice.

Simple and easy to understand

It started with a milk farmer. He had been referred to Keys for lumps on his eyelids and elbows. Upon examination, the lumps were found to contain pure cholesterol, a yellowish wax-like substance.

The farmer's cholesterol level was sky-high, at around TWENTY-FIVE. His brother's cholesterol was also high; they probably had a genetic defect.

Keys moved the brothers to his lab and fed them a completely fat-free diet (which wasn't very good) for a week, and their cholesterol level temporarily dropped. Keys had an idea. An idea that would have bigger repercussions.

There were two clues upon which Keys relied. In northern Europe, fewer people died from heart disease during the war when there was a shortage of food. Keys was very interested in the reason for that. The numbers implied that something we regularly ate, but of which there was a shortage during the war, resulted in heart disease. But what was it?

The second clue pertained to the trigger of heart disease. It starts with the tightening of arteries, created by a vascular blockage, or plaque. If the plaque ruptures, it will cause the blood to coagulate and create a scab inside the artery. That can clog up the artery so that the tissue on the other side dies due to the lack of oxygen and nutrition. If this occurs in the heart, it causes a heart attack. The plaque contains cholesterol.

The correlation was seemingly evident. The whole theory was very logical, at least to an engineer. Fatty food (later called saturated fat) caused the cholesterol in the blood to rise; the cholesterol was deposited in the arteries and caused heart disease. Had Keys found the solution?

They say every complicated problem has a simple answer that is easily misunderstood. The question is, whether or not Keys's theory was correct? There was only one way of finding out: to conduct a scientific test.

Seven countries

During the 1950s, Keys worked increasingly harder to clarify the correlation between fat, cholesterol, and heart disease. He examined the cholesterol levels of different groups of people, such as firefighters in Naples and rich and poor in Madrid.

He brought along his wife Margaret, who was a biochemist, to South Africa and let her do systematic tests of the cholesterol

Degenerative heart disease 1948–49, men aged 55–59.
Source: Keys A., 1953

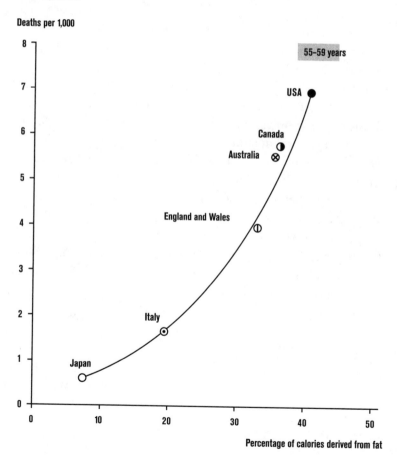

Deaths per 1,000

Percentage of calories derived from fat

levels among whites and blacks. Japan, Finland, Holland, Greece, Yugoslavia . . . Ancel Keys and his wife soon traveled around the world to examine cholesterol.

Keys believed he had found what he had been looking for. There seemed to be a correlation. Rich people and rich countries seemed to eat more fat and had higher cholesterol levels and frequency of heart disease.

He started to get more and more media attention. In an article from 1956, he is quoted saying: "The higher your income, the more fat you eat. But if you make more than $200 a week, you probably can't do more harm. You probably can't eat more fat."

It is here that the question marks start to appear in the story about Keys. Was he looking for the truth, or was he trying to prove that he was right?

If he was wrong, would he be able to admit it? In 1953, Keys published an investigation of the fat intake and frequency of heart disease in six countries (see the chart on the previous page). The more fat a country ate, the higher the frequency of heart disease. The correlation was remarkably evident. Judging from Keys's chart, the percentage of fat in one's food was the only thing that determined whether or not you would suffer from heart disease. Was it too good to be true? Yes, definitely.

A couple of years later, a skeptical colleague of Keys examined the research. Based on Keys's statistics, he produced the following chart (where each black dot corresponds to a country, some of which are labeled as examples):

Degenerative heart disease 1948–49, men aged 55–59

Source: Yerushalmy J, et al., 1957

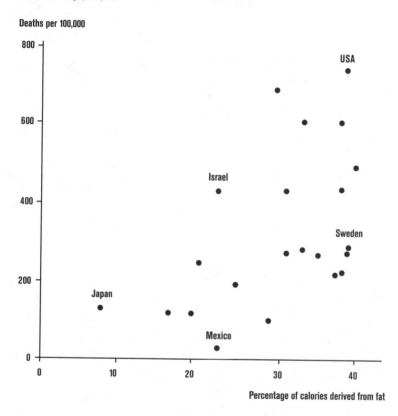

Deaths per 100,000

Percentage of calories derived from fat

There were actually figures available from twenty-two countries, not just the six that Keys had visited. Keys had managed to choose exactly those countries that illustrated maximum correlation.

To simply pick out the statistics that fit one's theory is a fatal scientific error. But the alleged forgery was not particularly well-known, and Keys was not backing down. He was already on his way to additional accomplishments, and he was well on his way to what many call his biggest contribution. The study that would become the main pillar of the fear of fat—the so-called Seven Countries study.

The study started in 1958 and followed twelve thousand middle-aged men in Italy, Greece, Yugoslavia, Holland, Finland, Japan, and the US They were monitored in terms of diet, cholesterol level, and if they suffered from heart disease. The study went on for decades and was impressively large for that time.

But here comes the second-to-most remarkable shift in the story. The Seven Countries study didn't even show a remote correlation between fat and heart disease. Not even a little bit. For example, in Greece (on Crete) they had eaten a lot of fat, but they actually had the fewest cases of heart disease.

This changed Keys's theory. It wasn't all types of fat that caused heart disease; it was a certain type of fat. The saturated fat. There was still a correlation between that and heart disease.[6] And this is where the fear of saturated fat began.

Fat for the warm-blooded

You might think that saturated fat sounds dangerous. So what is it? You can divide fat into two categories. Unsaturated fat is liquid at room temperature (like olive oil or sunflower oil). Saturated fat is solid at room temperature and can be found in animal fat (butter, lard) or tropical plants (coconut fat, palm oil).

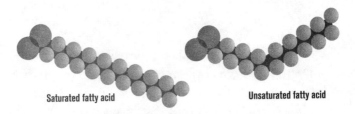

Saturated fatty acid   Unsaturated fatty acid

---

6. This is an ad hoc hypothesis, which was created as a retroactive explanation for when the original theory risked being proven wrong. These can often turn out to be right, but that is often a sign of an incorrect theory.

Ad hoc hypotheses are common within the pseudo-scientific community such as parapsychology. A funny example is how the advocates for biorhythmics were able to predict the gender of unborn babies. When an experiment turned out to be 50 percent successful, they said that the wrongly predicted babies probably included a lot of homosexuals.

Why is that? Don't worry, it is astonishingly simple. Fat consists of chains of carbon atoms (black in the images) with attached hydrogen atoms (gray).

Saturated fatty acids have an abundance of attached hydrogen atoms. Therefore, they are straight. If one or more hydrogen atoms are missing, the fatty acid becomes crooked. Depending on how many are missing, it becomes unsaturated or polyunsaturated.

Saturated (straight) fatty acids can be packed extra tight. That's why they turn solid at room temperature. But if they are heated, they separate from each other and become liquid. This is, for example, what happens when you heat butter in a saucepan.

What do you think is the most natural to eat? It is a trick question. Both are natural to eat.

You can find an abundance of saturated fat in the meat of all warm-blooded animals as well as in the milk of mammals. That is because saturated fat achieves the perfect consistency in body temperature, (i.e., 98.6 degrees Fahrenheit; 37 degrees Celsius). According to Ancel Keys, that kind of fat is dangerous for humans to consume. Those of us who are quick thinkers may see the obvious issue with such a statement.

Humans are warm-blooded animals. Our bodies are largely built from these types of fat and it can even be found in our breast milk. Then, how can it be poisonous? It is a strange idea. Could it be true?

Heart disease caused by municipal taxes

It doesn't really matter that Keys cheated to prove that he was right. Even if the studies had been conducted properly, they wouldn't have shown that fat correlates with heart disease. To think that it does indicates the same logical error that can be seen in tabloids every day. Here is one example: Could municipal taxes cause heart disease?

According to Keys's 1950s logic or today's tabloids, the answer is yes. Municipal taxation causes heart disease. See for yourself in the chart on the next page.

The correlation between heart disease and municipal taxation

Source: Uffe Ravnskov, Fat and cholesterol are healthier by Optimal Publishing 2008, p.29.

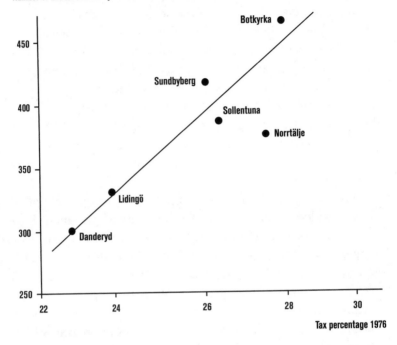

Number of deaths caused by heart attacks per 100,000

Botkyrka

450

Sundbyberg

400

Sollentuna

Norrtälje

350

Lidingö

300

Danderyd

250

22   24   26   28   30

Tax percentage 1976

In municipalities with high taxes, many people die from heart disease. In municipalities with low taxes, people are healthier. Could it be more self-evident?

Think one step further. Elongate the curve to the left. Then you'll see that if municipal taxes decrease to 9 percent, no one will die from heart disease any longer.

Everyone knows that logic is flawed. The correlation has to stem from something else. Perhaps wealthier municipalities with lower on average taxes have healthier inhabitants. The example seems silly. But the point is that it is the exact same type of chart as in Keys's research about fat consumption and heart disease. We have simply switched out the amount of fat intake to tax percentage. The difference is that the correlation *feels* more reasonable.

From a scientific standpoint, the evidence for a real correlation is weak. Statistical correlation does not prove causation.

It is the same problem we experience with tabloid headlines which repeatedly claim that x causes y; for example "poor air quality leads to obesity" or "you become thinner by eating breakfast." However, the fact that poorer and heavier people live in regions with more pollution does not prove that the air affected their weight. The fact that thin people on average have regular breakfast habits does not prove that you lose weight from eating more food.

Observational studies where you study what people do and see what happens do not prove causation. They simply provide a theory that needs to be corroborated with other methods.

Another example: the more ice cream Swedes eat, the more people drown. The correlation is clear. Does that prove eating ice cream makes you drown? Or does the cause depend on something else, such as the fact that both events are common in the summertime?[7]

Even if it wasn't necessary for Ancel Keys to doctor his research, he needed proof of the harmfulness of fat similar to the proof that showed that ice cream causes people to drown. Since he only selected countries that fit his theory, the proof was even less legitimate.

There are good reasons why we still discuss what kind of food is healthy in the long run. That is because it is difficult for modern science to determine it with absolute certainty. A fair study is not only difficult to conduct, but it is also devastatingly expensive and time-consuming.

What you need is an "intervention study" where an enormously large group of people is divided into two groups. One group is advised to eat as little fat as possible and the other to eat more thereof. The groups should then be closely monitored for a long period of time that would account for statistical biases such as diseases and death. Perhaps

---

7. The examples are endless. A fun observational study, conducted as a joke, apparently showed that heart disease was caused by something completely different—whether or not you have a beard. It is apparently more common for people who rarely shave to be afflicted by heart disease. The more seldom a person shaves, the more that person gets heart complications.

Before you unnecessarily shave off your beard: the correlation probably stems from something else. Can you guess what?

even for a decade, if there are tens of thousands of participants. If the difference is clear, that is the answer. Did the theory about the danger of fat turn out to be true or not?

A random intervention study is fair, since it is only one thing that sets the two groups apart. In observational studies, thousands of things differ and it is impossible to attribute causation. In intervention studies, you know that since one thing separates the participants, that must be the cause.

In the beginning of the 1970s, the United States considered conducting such an experiment. The problem? It was expected to cost $1.3 billion USD. No one wanted to foot the bill. Instead they decided to launch a couple of smaller, cheaper studies. They would also take a decade to complete, and it was unclear whether or not they would prove anything. Not everyone wanted to just wait and see.

Selling one's theory

What happened to the second theory, the one about sugar and starch causing Western diseases? In the middle of the twentieth century, wealthy countries that suffered from heart diseases didn't just consume more saturated fat. The same connection could be made to sugar and white flour. Cleave, the outsider, had quietly highlighted the connection to many new diseases, but the main contention would arise around cardiovascular disease. Which was the culprit—fat or sugar?

The two theories were mirror images of each other, and both could hardly be true. One would have to go so the other one could shine. That meant there was another internationally renowned scientist that stood in Ancel Keys's way.

Professor John Yudkin was born in 1910 and grew up in London, in a poor Jewish family that had escaped the oppression in Russia. In the 1930s, he married a Jewish woman who had fled from Germany and they spent the rest of their lives together.

After serving as a military doctor in West Africa, he became a professor in physiology at London University. Yudkin's research during the next few decades shows that sugar had a strong connection to heart disease. He later wrote the book *Pure, White, and Deadly*. The title was of course referring to sugar.

John Yudkin was convinced that the theory about the dangers of fat was incorrect, and that sugar and carbohydrates were the culprits. Ancel Keys was convinced of the opposite. The world was not big enough for the both of them. Who would emerge victorious?

If Yudkin was right, Keys had made a mistake and all his work would have been for naught. Unsurprisingly, Ancel Keys was ruthless in his determination.

Keys composed a long letter, uncharacteristically filled with spite, in which he went into detail about why Yudkin's research was worthless. He sent the letter to all prominent experts on the area and published it in a major medical journal. He claimed that it was absurd of Yudkin to use statistics from forty-one countries to prove a correlation between sugar consumption and heart disease. Keys never mentioned the fact that he himself had used the same statistics, but from only six countries, to strengthen his theory about fat.

It got worse. Yudkin was not a particularly good public speaker, so when he debated Ancel Keys, he usually lost. The fight against Keys did not end well. It probably didn't help that Yudkin also managed to make the sugar industry his enemy.

Yudkin retired early in 1971 and his university replaced him with someone who believed in the dangerous nature of fat. Yudkin moved to Israel. Keys had obliterated his credibility. Anyone who later claimed to doubt that fat was dangerous could easily be dismissed as being "just like Yudkin." A condescending term with a threatening tone. People were about to conform.

Yudkin ended his days in ridicule and dismissed as a joke. He was never vindicated. But one question remains: was Yudkin right? If they had known in the 1970s what was about to happen, he would not have been dismissed as easily.[8]

The submissive alternative

The theory about the danger of fat was about to become common knowledge. Professor Yudkin and the dangers of sugar had been dismissed. So what was going to happen to all of the stories about populations that had become sicker during the decades following the arrival of the new sugar and white flour—Cleave's theory? A theory that could be as potentially world-changing as that of the theory of antibiotics? It needed to be explained away.

The problem was essentially very simple. If fat was dangerous, carbohydrates had to be healthy. Otherwise there would be nothing with which to replace the fat.

Doctor Denis Burkitt made two large contributions throughout his career. First time around, he was right. He worked as a surgeon in Africa during the 1950s and was the first person to describe a very special kind of cancer, one caused by a virus. The cancer was later named Burkitt lymphoma. He had made something out of himself, so people listened to him.

Back in England, he was introduced to Cleave, whose theory he found to be brilliant and extremely important. Burkitt wrote the foreword for Cleave's book *The Saccharine Disease*. But Burkitt's second contribution was a complete distortion of the theory that ended up sabotaging it.

Burkitt knew that Cleave was right. When he visited hospitals in the United States, he saw tons of obese African-Americans with diabetes and heart disease. These conditions barely existed in Africa, where Burkitt had worked. The disease appeared to correlate with

---

8. Some people exist before their time. Rober H. Lustig from San Francisco, who studies this topic, celebrated Yudkin in his now famous 2009 lecture. It has over half a million hits on YouTube: "Sugar: The Bitter Truth."

 Lustig talks about how "every detail [Yudkin] predicted has occurred. It is astonishing. I am extremely impressed by him."

the sugar and white flour. But did the problem arise from something in the new food—or something that was missing?

Denis Burkitt, like an astonishing number of people back then, was obsessed with constipation. The more Western food that was consumed, like sugar and white flour, the more fiber one consumed and the more feces were produced. Less feces means a slower intestinal process, which Burkitt believed was the cause of our modern diseases.

He experimented on his family to observe the time it took for something that was swallowed to reach the other side. Soon he repeated the experiment with 1,200 volunteers in different parts of the world.

He measured the time it took for food to pass through the digestive system and the fecal texture. In Uganda, the record was 2.2 lbs (980 g) of feces per day. The Brits could barely produce a fraction of that, and constipation was a common ailment.[9]

Burkitt inverted Cleave's theory. He claimed that the problem was not the purified carbohydrates, but rather the lack of the fibers that had been removed. The advantage was obvious. The theory could suddenly coexist with the theory about the dangers of fat. That was its major breakthrough. A low-fat and fiber-rich diet became synonymous with healthy food. Does that sound familiar?

The problem with Burkitt's transformation of Cleave's theory is simple. It is incorrect. The lack of fiber could never explain the arrival of the new Western diseases. They never afflicted populations that ate minimal amounts of fiber and carbohydrates, such as the Inuit, Eskimos, or the Massai and Sami people. They were healthy without fiber. It was not until the arrival of sugar and the white flour that they became ill. The fiber theory couldn't explain it.

Since Burkitt's heydays, plenty of studies have tested fiber's effect on preventing all types of diseases. Time after time they have produced negative results. The only thing on which fiber actually seems to have an impact is constipation. Otherwise, it mostly seems to

---

9. Denis Burkitt's interest in the subject seems to have been limitless. He used to say that the health of the population could be predicted by the volume of their feces, and the fluctuation thereof. One time he even managed to shock a very tough crowd of gastroenterologists by asking whether or not they knew the "size of their wife's feces."

produce gas and stomach aches within sensitive people. Fibers also impair the absorption of carbohydrates, which is positive. But without sugar and starch, you don't seem to need extra fiber.

Cleave and Yudkin were extremely close to the truth. But toward the end of the 1970s, their research was about to be forgotten. It was about to collect dust for the next couple of decades. Instead, we were about to see the consequences of doing the complete opposite.

Politicians determine things

It was difficult to scientifically determine whether or not sugar was possibly dangerous. But in some areas, it became increasingly popular. The spirit of the 1970s helped. Meat and eggs were seen as an exploitation of Earth's resources, and a vegetarian, low-fat diet was considered the solution to starvation in Africa.

While research remained ambiguous, the evidence nonexistent, and the theories divided, the winner was about to be selected in an unconventional way.

The scene was a political committee in the United States, led by Senator George McGovern. They had handled the issue of malnutrition, which had started to be resolved. But before they concluded the decision, they had to review the problem of over-nutrition.

In July 1976, after two days of testimonials from experts, they wrote the first edition of *The Diet of the United States*. When it came down to fat, they predominantly relied on the experts that were convinced of the dangerous nature of fat, and the recommendation was to reduce one's fat consumption.

When the report was released in January 1977, all hell broke loose. The low-fat recommendations were extremely controversial and many were against them. McGovern called the committee to a meeting and made them listen to a lecture from the experts. Many experts claimed that advice about reduced fat intake was pure speculation, without demonstrated utility, and with an obvious risk of unknown side effects. Other experts offered their support.

They later published an updated version of the official dietary recommendations with more relaxed phrasing, but with a similar low-fat theme. The controversy continued for years to come. A low-fat diet gradually became the norm.

The scientific world was still in deep disagreement about the benefit of reduced fat. But that was about to change.

The hunt for evidence

Starting a definitive American study for the price of $1.245 million would have been deemed too expensive. Instead, they launched six smaller studies to prove the dangers of fat. The results came in, one by one, during the 1980s.

Unfortunately, the first five studies could not demonstrate a correlation between fat intake and heart disease. The largest study, MRFIT, had cost over $142 million. Participants received help to quit smoking and blood-pressure medication, in addition to being recommended a low-fat diet. Despite this, there were no evident improvements to their hearts.

There was a problem. Many people were sure fat was dangerous, and the official dietary recommendations had already started spreading the message. The only thing missing was evidence. But evidence was difficult to come by. Despite having spent millions of dollars in this hunt, there was no sure evidence to prove their theory right.

Eventually it arrived—that which would change most people's minds and shut the rest up. It was neither a food study nor low-fat diets. It was cholesterol—a study of cholesterol reduction through medicine.

The last of the six studies produced the long-awaited results: statistically significant numbers. Indeed it was not a dietary study; it was a study about medicine, but sometimes you have to run with what you get.

The study tested a cholesterol-reducing medicine on men with extremely high cholesterol levels. The risk of dying from a heart attack during the study was somewhat lower than in the medication group: 1.6 percent compared to 2 percent in the control group.

So, the study was testing a medication. But the conclusion was that a low-fat diet would produce the same cholesterol-reducing results. That was something the study had not even tested, something that every similar study has failed to this day.

In the absence of real proof, they took a chance. After all, most people were already convinced that the theory about the dangers of fat was correct. People died from heart attacks every day and no one wanted to wait for more studies. There were essentially no other studies going on at the time, and new ones would take many years. It was time to take action.[10]

Agriculture (more starch) and the industrial revolution (sugar, white flour) were the first two transformations of humanity's diet. During our historical year, we have reached the midnight countdown on New Year's Eve and the third and last transformation.

The year was 1984. A massive campaign was launched to teach the American population to be scared of fat and cholesterol.

Putting everything on red

The theory that all the new things in humans' diets—sugar and white flour—were behind our Western diseases had been dismissed. That happened before any high-quality studies were done, despite the fact that smaller studies had shown positive results.

The sugar and starch theory would go on to live in the periphery of "real" science, with an aura of being an alternative medicine. First and foremost as an effective but highly controversial weight loss diet. The theory was no longer welcome in the nicer areas of society.

---

10. Do you want to read more about how the theory about the dangers of fat arose? I can recommend the award-winning American science journalist Gary Taube's writing.

In 2001, Taube started with the article "The Soft Science of Dietary Fat" in the journal *Science* and followed up with the acclaimed "What if it's all been a Big Fat Lie?" in the *New York Times* in 2002. These articles can be read online; just search online for the titles. Thereafter, Taube spent five years writing the book *Good Calories, Bad Calories*, which was published in 2007. It is a fantastic book about the history and science around food and health, although it is a very thick book.

Sooner or later it was time to decide for certain. In 1984 it was time to comply and for scientists to focus all their energy on a joint cause. The winner of the two competing theories had been selected, and that was the theory about the dangers of fat.

The winner was chosen during an official "consensus conference." The board was comprised of people who were already convinced. Dissidents did not affect the conclusion. There were "no doubts," they said, that a low-fat diet would protect Americans older than two years against heart disease.

Stubborn dissidents were ostracized. If you wanted federal funding for your research, you had to stick to approved research, or finance it yourself. Dietary research that followed was based on the premise that fat increased cholesterol, which in turn resulted in heart disease.

Skeptics were not favored. One example is Uffe Ravnskov, a Danish physician and scientist who had worked in Sweden and lives in Lund. The more he studied the issue, the more holes he found in the theory about the dangers of fat. He went on to write the book *The Cholesterol Myth*, which was harshly criticized. It was literally set on fire on Finnish TV. Ravnskov has later discussed how proud he was when he heard that. He was thrilled to be among the authors who have had one of their books burnt.

It would take decades before Ravnskov and other skeptics would come out somewhat on top. That is because they had scientific reasons to be doubtful.

But in 1984, there were no doubts. Scientists' official world view was set in more or less solid stone. Fat and saturated fat increased cholesterol levels, and cholesterol produced heart attacks. The fat had to go. The message was simple, very simple: America was going to eat less fat.

Naturally, fatty food had become a "greasy killer," as one interest group put it. The food industry was quick to see the economic opportunities. Grocery stores stocked up on low-fat products with less fat and cheaper starch and sugar. Even soda, sports drinks, and juice—sugar solutions—would look healthy.

After all, soda is 100 percent fat-free.

The epidemic

All in all, you could say society took a chance without ascertaining evidence, despite the fact that famous scientists warned that there might be unforeseen dangerous consequences. Never before had an entire population received the advice to avoid fat. No one could know what was going to happen. It was an experiment.

In retrospect, we could have suspected a risk. If you avoid fat, you eat more carbohydrates, more of the new food, sugar and white flour, which increases the blood sugar and insulin levels, the body's fat-storing hormone.

More carbohydrates, more insulin, more obesity. That risk was dismissed. But that is what happened. The result was evident only a couple of years later. Today, a couple of decades later, the discrepancy is enormous.

The official obesity statistics from the United States are staggering. Suddenly, from having been consistent throughout the 1960s and 1970s at around 13 percent, something changed in the middle of the 1980s. The curve spiked and kept rising.

It has been incredibly fast. It quickly passed 15 percent obesity, then 20 and 25 percent obese Americans, and now it's 30 percent, and approaching 35 percent. That is a tripling of the number of obese people in one single generation.[11] The number of overweight and obese people combined amount to 68 percent.

Obesity has taken over in the United States in an unprecedented way. Now the epidemic is spreading across the Western world and beyond.

The term "average weight" loses its meaning when not even every third American has a normal weight, and that number keeps decreasing. That raises a question that might actually have an answer. When will *all* Americans be overweight or obese? When will the last thin American be history?

---

11. A normal weight is a BMI between 18.5-24.9; overweight >25; obesity >30. One's BMI is calculated by squaring the product of one's weight divided by one's height.

The question is not unreasonable. Scientists have attempted to calculate it. The answer? If the trend continues, there will be no average-weight Americans by 2048.

It gets worse. Along with obesity, a diabetes epidemic has spread across the world. And obesity and diabetes is only the visible top of the iceberg. Under the surface we find the rest of Western diseases that are the root of our endemic diseases.

Sweden follows suit

The United States did not keep their dietary recommendations to themselves. They spread to the rest of the Western world, including Sweden, which also received the advice to avoid fat. The Swedish symbol for this fear—the keyhole mark—arrived in 1989. (The keyhole is a Nordic nutrition label that makes it easier for consumers to choose food that contains less fat, salt, and sugar, and more whole grain and fiber.)

Since the 1980s, Sweden was increasingly warned about the dangers of eating fatty food, and warned about the naturally saturated fat. The most dangerous and evil fat was butter. Sales therefore plummeted.

The low-fat diet would not only make us healthier. In theory it contained fewer calories. That's why it would also make us thinner, they said. But that didn't happen. Instead, the opposite happened—in Sweden as well as in the United States.

If you compare official statistics of overweight and obese Swedes with butter sales, you find an interesting contrast: As soon as people started worrying about fat, obesity gained traction. The more we avoided fat, the heavier we became. Something was very wrong. More and more people are starting to question things. During the 2000s, Swedes have started to discuss and doubt the low-fat dietary recommendation. Butter sales have started to rise again. At the same time, the rise of obesity has stagnated.

Obesity and butter sales in Sweden 1980-2009

Source: SCB:s ULF-studies 1980-2002, NIH health survey 2004-2009 and Swedish milk

Butter sales (tons/year)

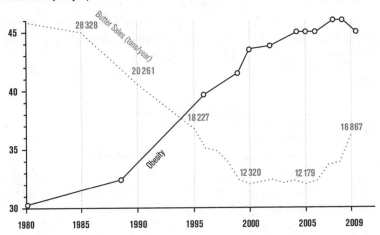

Today

If we are getting more obese using today's dietary recommendations, what would happen if we did the complete opposite? Modern studies have shown exciting results.

Proof of the theory about the dangers of fat didn't exist in 1984. What about today? The scientific community is more divided than ever. That becomes increasingly evident every year. Something is about to happen. The defense of the old is fading away. The alternative is gaining traction.

The only thing that maintains the status quo is the ingrained belief that natural fat causes heart disease. If that belief doesn't hold true, everything will come tumbling down. Then everything can change. And now, something is happening. A new paradigm. A revolution.

It's happening here and now.

CHAPTER THREE

The demise of the world as we know it

They have been bugging us about low-fat diets for thirty years and then it turns out to be completely wrong! There is no proof of a correlation between saturated fat and heart disease.

FREDRIK NYSTRÖM
Professor of internal medicine, Linköping University Hospital

S weden is pioneering this. The scientific revolution that is taking place across the globe is starting to blossom. The results could have unimaginable consequences.

Let's take a step back again. What do I mean that something is about to happen? To understand this we need scientific theory. Don't worry, we won't get into too much detail, even if it's surprisingly interesting.

In 1962, when Thomas Kuhn wrote the book *The Structure of Scientific Revolutions*, he became the most influential scientific theorist in modern history. He presented a new idea about how scientific progress is made: usually slowly but surely, one piece of the puzzle at a time. But sometimes, the opposite is true. More and more pieces no longer fit into the puzzle, no matter how hard you try. Eventually the contradictions became too many to ignore and explain away. A revolution is inevitable.

The revolution is a paradigm shift. Scientists always interpret their research area from their current perception of the world, their paradigm. In revolutions, the old world view is thrown out. A new and better perspective takes over. A new way of piecing together the puzzle. A clearer picture, in which all of the pieces fit together.

In the beginning of the seventeenth century, Earth was the obvious center of the universe. All astronomers knew this to be true. The sun and the planets revolved around Earth, period. Unfortunately, it was for some reason difficult to predict the movement of planets in that way.

Copernicus and Galileo Galilei realized that there was a better way of explaining things: Earth and the planets all revolve around the sun. We now know that they were right. But the resistance against changing common knowledge was strong.

Copernicus was discreet, but Galilei was not. In 1633 we saw a heretic convicted by the church. He was placed under house arrest for the rest of his life and was deprived of books. But the scientific revolution could not be stopped in the long run. Earth is not the center of the universe. Earth revolves around the sun. The old world view eventually eroded.

During the nineteenth century, no one wanted to believe that diseases could stem from the spread of infectious bacteria. Everyone knew that diseases appeared randomly out of nothing, often from bad air or miasma. Therefore, there were no valid reasons why doctors should wash their hands. That was incorrect, and countless people died in vain from cholera and postpartum infection before bacteria theory had its breakthrough.

World view changes in science happen now and then. It is not a strange thing. On the contrary, they are sometimes inevitable. They can happen violently. There could arise an intellectual battle between early adopters and those who stick to the old truth. If the new world view is sufficiently better, it eventually becomes dogma. But it takes years or sometimes decades before the switch is complete.

Mahatma Gandhi's classic quote describes how a shift can take place from the perspective of the early adopters: "First they ignore you, then they laugh at you, then they fight you, then you win."

Not everyone is keen on changing his or her world view, despite how clear the evidence is. They say that a new scientific theory breaks through not by proving dissenters wrong and making them see the light, but because they eventually die out. A new generation who knows the new theory takes over.

It might sound unnecessarily dramatic. But the fact is that people have a difficult time embracing new things when they have spent their whole careers teaching others something that is incorrect. That takes a very big person.

It can be difficult to admit "I was wrong" about little things. When it comes to something on which you have built your whole career, that can be difficult to admit even to yourself. Few can handle it.[12]

The Titanic and the iceberg

What does this mean for the science of food and your health? As in many other areas, even these scientists and doctors have a world view, a paradigm. And it is slowly eroding. The revolution has gained traction.

The main theory has been evident for decades. "Saturated fat raises cholesterol" and "high cholesterol causes heart disease." The low-fat model was for healthy food. It infected other similar areas.

Suddenly, without evidence, low-fat food filled with insulin-raising carbohydrates was the best way of losing weight. A few decades later, the world is heavier than ever.

Suddenly, without evidence, low-fat food filled with blood sugar-raising carbohydrates was the best thing a diabetic could eat. A few decades later, we find ourselves in the midst of an

---

12. It is a well-known phenomenon. Leo Tolstoy, the nineteenth-century Russian writer, described it as:

"I know that most men, including those at ease with problems of the greatest complexity, can seldom accept even the simplest and most obvious truth if it be such as would oblige them to admit the falsity of conclusions which they have delighted in explaining to colleagues, which they have proudly taught to others, and which they have woven, thread by thread, into the fabric of their lives."

The actual diet debate offers some astonishing examples of this.

unprecedented diabetes epidemic where the sick become sicker and more people require medicines.

Something is obviously wrong. But reality is not the main reason for today's crisis. That requires something bigger, namely science. Despite its flaws, many perceived the theory about the dangers of fat as unsinkable. Like the Titanic. But it crashed into its own massive iceberg on February 8, 2006.

That day, by far the largest study on the subject was published by the Women's Health Initiative. It was a study that had cost $700 million American tax dollars and had been conducted over the course of eight years, which would demonstrate the utility of what they had done for decades, namely scaring the population away from fat. The result was not what they had hoped; far from it, in fact.

Fifty thousand women were randomly split into two groups. The control group was asked to keep on living normally. The other received intensive help to reduce their fat intake and eat more fruit and greens. In a total of forty-six instances, specialized dieticians educated them on what to eat and why they should eat less fat. It worked. They ate more fruit and greens. They even exercised more than the control group.

Tens of thousands of women struggled with low-fat products and avoided fat. Did they turn out healthier? In 2006, the answer came in black and white. The answer was no. The participants who had kept a low-fat diet did not have fewer instances of cancer. They did not have less heart disease. They had not become healthier at all.

That in and of itself seems to suggest that we have eaten low-fat products with sugar and additives in vain. Like Karin Bojs, journalist and director at the leading Swedish newspaper *Dagens Nyheter* (The Daily News) wrote: "The findings of the Women's Health Initiatives is the last nail in the coffin for the old dogma 'eat less fat.'"

But it gets worse. Was the low-fat diet just unnecessary for your health, or did it in fact have a negative impact? The study included a couple thousand women with heart disease. If a low-fat diet positively impacts heart disease, it should be evident among those with a heart condition. Those women actually got worse from the low-fat diet!

This fantastic finding was excluded from the summary. It's not even included in the summarizing table. Interestingly, out of forty-three results, one has vanished. That's the result for those with a heart precondition. Truly something that would delight any conspiracy theorist.

To see how people with a heart condition became sicker from a low-fat diet, you have to read the fine print of the results. But it is in there. You can easily read it yourself, stuck in a paragraph on the seventh page of the study.[13] A low-fat diet provided a 26 percent increased risk for people with a heart condition to suffer from a heart attack or stroke. That is statistically significant. The cover-up was highlighted in a comment of the study, which was published in a later edition.

If this result is true, it is astounding. It means that people with a heart condition who have followed the recommendation to keep a low-fat diet haven't just been doing so in vain. They have even become significantly sicker from it.

The fact that such a spectacular finding, the only significant one in the whole study, was hidden away can only be explained in one way. It was too much. The researchers were already disappointed that their large study had failed to verify what they set out to prove. The fact that it could be the complete opposite was against their entire world view. It could only be seen as an embarrassing and unlikely coincidence.

It probably wasn't a coincidence. That is clearer today. The low-fat diet hit its iceberg with this study, by far the largest one around. It shocked many back then. But in the last couple of years, three major reviews of the research have given us the answer sheet. The results are starting to become common knowledge. More and more people are embracing the facts.

We will return to the sinking theory about the dangers of fat later. To see something so large sink is very exciting. Hearing the orchestra, the Swedish equivalent to the USDA pretends that noth-

---

13. In the reference section in the back of the book, there are citations for all studies mentioned in the text. Many, including this one, can be read for free by anyone with an Internet connection.

ing is happening while the captivating truth is slowly surfacing. But first, how could we be so easily fooled?

Science v. Mother Nature

With the beauty of hindsight, it is difficult to understand how we could fall for the theory about the dangers of fat. Still, even I believed it, despite how unbelievable that might sound today. Because how could saturated fat in butter or meat be dangerous?

Like with all warm-blooded animals, your body is mostly comprised of saturated fat. It has an appropriate consistency at body temperature.

It is a stable kind of fat that doesn't easily go rancid. Humans have always consumed saturated fat, such as meat or eggs. Breast milk is filled with saturated fat. Your brain is predominantly built from saturated fats. Every cell in your body needs saturated fat to construct the protective cell membrane. Saturated fat is good fat.

The madness is clearest in today's food advice for infants. According to the Swedish USDA, all children, regardless of age or weight, should only be fed low-fat milk, from the day they stop breastfeeding. Anything else is perceived as bad for the child's cholesterol levels. There's only one problem. Breast milk is almost ten times fattier than low-fat milk, most of which is actually saturated fat. If saturated fat was dangerous, breastfeeding mothers would be poisoning their children.

There is one additional problem with the theory. The more natural fat one removes, the more consistency, color, and flavor additives are required for something to appear as normal food.

Recently, a blog held a contest to discover the product that contained the most e-numbers [EU food additives]. The winner? Rydbergs Low-Fat Skagenröra, Swedish shrimp mixed together with crème fraîche, caviar, and dill. Among many things, it contained stabilizers (E407, E412, E413, E415, E460, E466, E1414, E1422), preservatives (E202, E211), coloring (E104, E120, E16A, E170, E171), acid (E270, E296, E300, E330), and flavor enhancements (E575, E621, E627, E631). Perhaps it contained some little shrimp among the total of twenty-three e-numbers. It is difficult to believe that these types of chemistry sets could be healthier than real food.

Since 1989, the keyhole nutrition label is supposed to "make it easier for the consumer to choose healthy food." But the label first and foremost means that the product follows the old recommendation about less fat and saturated fat. It is thus nothing to worry about today.

Keyhole-labeled low-fat products usually contain more additives than food with natural fat. Rarely are they healthier than the food they are replacing. You can still find keyhole-marked low-fat yogurts that have been deprived of almost all natural fat but that contain so much added sugar that a liter sometimes contains 90 grams thereof. That is almost the same sugar level as soda. How can you call keyhole-labeled candy healthy? There should be a better way of conducting public health work.

Why do low-fat products taste worse? Why do they all need these flavor enhancers? Well, saturated fat is an excellent carrier of flavor that brings out other flavors in food. Saturated fats, such as butter, make food taste better. Ask any chef.

In 2009, the Swedish chef team received a sponsorship from Unilever for a record-short period of time. It is a chemistry company that, among many things, produces fake butter like the margarine brand Promise. They are made from cheap vegetable oils with less saturated fat. The national chef team was supposed to demonstrate how you can cook good food with margarine.

The sponsorship was a fiasco. As major Swedish newspaper *Svenska Dagbladet* wrote, "Talk about bad will and a failed collaboration . . . this has to be one of the private sector's worst sponsorship attempts." The national chef team refused the sponsorship. "Everyone knows that chefs cook with butter," one chef stated. Another said what he really thought: "I wash my clothes with their laundry detergent . . . their low-fat food products are garbage, in my opinion."

We have unnecessarily been afraid of natural and good food. It has been traded for tasteless low-fat products filled with additives and sugar. Things that can really make you obese and sick. But the confusion is getting closer to its end.

A transparent smoke screen

Thousands of studies from the past fifty years pertain to the utility of fat or the dangers thereof. It is easy to hand-pick uncertain studies with fitting messages and claim that they in general demonstrate that saturated fat is detrimental. That is what advocates for the theory of fat have done for decades. So what's the problem? This is not how you conduct serious research to find the truth. In the absence of evidence, they are producing a smoke screen.

Depending on how you pick and interpret small studies on the subject, you could claim that saturated fat is healthy, unhealthy, or neither. That's simple. But it doesn't prove anything and leads nowhere.

In 2009, the Swedish USDA offered a funny example. They tried to defend its dietary recommendations from the increasingly harsh criticism. The agency produced a list where seventy-two studies claimed to demonstrate that saturated fat was dangerous, whereas only eight proved its innocence.

The list quickly became a joke. It was not an effective smoke screen. It was completely transparent. In *Today's Medicine*, the list was analyzed by twelve professors and doctors. One of them was Lars Werkö, a professor and an icon within Swedish healthcare.

Of the seventy-two studies that were claimed to show the dangers of saturated fat, eleven did not even talk about saturated fat. A couple of them actually said that saturated fat was healthy. It was a concoction of uncertain studies that didn't really show anything. The review determined that the list and the warnings against saturated fat "lacked any credibility."

The Swedish USDA met the critique with an extremely evasive response which didn't even mention saturated fat. The spectacle finished when the editor-in-chief at *Today's Medicine* stated what many were thinking concerning the diet debate: "The Swedish

USDA is escaping responsibility." Its strategy is "unintelligible" and refusing to answer "is not credible."

I don't think that the Swedish USDA's strategy is unintelligible. They did what they could to avoid losing face. They actually still have problems to this day.

There is only one way to prove that the theory about the dangers of fat is correct. You would have to conduct a study that really proves that people become healthier from eating less fat. What you need is a randomized intervention study with hard endpoints.

The participants are split into two groups, which constitutes the "randomization." One group keeps a low-fat diet while the other doesn't. Then you track the participants for a significant period of time to record any instances of disease or death. Such health effects are "hard endpoints." It is simply not enough to show a difference in a blood sample that is difficult to interpret. You have to demonstrate a true effect on people's health.

Such studies are required to demonstrate, for example, that a medication has an effect. Nowadays it is virtually impossible to legally sell a painkiller without showing one or preferably multiple studies.

How many high-quality studies of the like do you think they have shown in order to be able to recommend a "healthy" low-fat diet to the entire population?

Hundreds? Ten? Do you think there is a single one? Astonishingly enough, the correct answer is zero. There is not one high-quality study verifying that saturated fat is dangerous.

You can play an entertaining game with professors and others who believe in the theory of the dangers of fat. Ask if they know of such a study, and they often say yes. They probably take for granted that one exists. Then ask for a specific example. It is not strange that they have a difficult time responding. There is no answer.

The lack of evidence has not gone unnoticed by everyone. The Swedish Heart and Lung Foundation previously sponsored the margarine brand Promise with "millions of Swedish crowns." That gave Promise the right to feature the Foundation's symbol on its packaging. In February 2009, the Swedish Heart and Lung Foundation terminated the collaboration and said no to the margarine money. The reason was that modern studies showed that switching to margarine isn't necessarily healthy. "The scientific basis for the dangers of saturated fat is pretty weak," as the foundation's information director Roger Höglund carefully expressed it.

There is not one single piece of evidence that supports the theory about the dangers of fat. Only one thing remains. Blowing the smoke screen away.

Game over

How do you solve the issue that all of these small studies point toward opposite conclusions and can essentially support any opinion out there? How do you blow away the smoke so that you can uncover the truth?

The answer is a systematic review of all the studies. A review where you do not simply hand-pick studies that fit your preconceived notions, but one that reviews everything. That would be a huge undertaking. Recently, three research groups have tried to tackle it.

The first group was led by Andre Mente, a Canadian professor. They reviewed every single relevant study from 1950 and onward, over five thousand of them. In April of 2009, their findings were published in the renowned scientific journal *Archives of Internal Medicine*. The results were clear. There was "insufficient evidence" to prove that the total fat intake, saturated fat, polyunsaturated fat, meat, egg, or dairy have anything to do with heart disease.

It can be difficult to embrace such news. But more and more people are doing so. In September of 2009, Fredrik Nyström, professor of internal medicine, said: "They have been bugging us about low-fat diets for thirty years and then it turns out to be completely wrong! There is no proof of a correlation between saturated fat and heart disease."

What does that mean for you? You can comfortably eat butter and drink cream if you so wish. That is completely safe if we are to believe this extensive review of all studies. But to make sure, let's hear it from other sources.

The other review was part of a large report published by the World Health Organization (WHO) in September 2009. It showed the same results. People who eat less fat or saturated fat do not become healthier, in neither observational studies nor in more certain controlled studies.

A group led by the researcher Siri-Tarino conducted the third review. It was published in January 2010 in the scientific journal *American Journal of Clinical Nutrition*, perhaps the most renowned journal in the world of nutritional science.

They add all the quality observational studies that had examined how much saturated fat people consume and how healthy they are. Around twenty or so studies, comprising a total of over 300,000 people who had been tracked for decades, were added together.

The results? There is no correlation between saturated fat intake and heart disease. People who eat a lot of saturated fat do not become sicker than people who keep a low-fat diet.

Peter M. Nilsson, professor of cardiovascular research, recently spoke in front of five hundred doctors at a big conference in Stockholm. He summarized it like this: "This means we have to put an end to this. There is no correlation between saturated fat intake and cardiovascular disease."

Could it be clearer? Perhaps like this: game over.

The paradigm is shifting

Is it time to appoint an official government commission of inquiry?

We can no longer avoid the suspicion. Have the misguided recommendations led to a disaster? More people are thinking the same thought. The paradigm shift is underway. Johan Frostengård, professor of medicine at Karolinska Institutet, recently said: "We have underestimated the risks of carbohydrates and overestimated the dangers of fat."

More and more people are refusing to wait for permission from some slow government agency. Many have already realized that it is time to abandon the sinking ship. There is no health reason today to eat low-fat products with additives and added sugar. An increasing number of Swedes eat fatty food again. Butter sales are on the rise again.

The letters to the editor sections and journalistic reports repeatedly tell a familiar story. After having become fat and sick when they tried to follow the low-fat dietary recommendations, many people are now becoming thinner and healthier when they do the complete opposite.

Swedes have debated diets for years. These diets range from: eating natural food without additives, which excludes low-fat products—to alternative diets that don't have such a fear of fat, such as GI (avoiding sugar and simple carbohydrates) and LCHF (avoiding the majority of carbohydrates). Now something fantastic could be about to happen. The worldwide obesity epidemic that gained traction in the 1980s seems to be rising to new levels across the globe, everywhere, in all countries—with one exception.

During the twenty-first century, the Swedish obesity epidemic has slowed down. There has been no increase the last couple of years and the latest numbers point toward a change. At the very least, it seems like children, and perhaps women, are becoming leaner again. Sweden has started the revolution. The debate has only begun in some parts of the rest of the world, whereas in Sweden it has been around for years among the general population. Perhaps it is on its way to making us thin again. Perhaps we'll be the first country in the world to reverse this epidemic.

While Sweden might have stagnated and is turning around the trend of about 12 percent obese adults, the United States is continuing toward the abyss. In the US, where the fear of being overweight began, people are now scared to death of anything with "fat" in it. Grocery stores are filled with Low Fat and No Fat. It can be difficult to find any real food whatsoever. But it hasn't made them thin; quite the opposite. Now an astounding 34 percent of Americans are obese and just as many are overweight.

Why should we uncritically follow the Americans' way toward disaster?

Like Albert Einstein once said: "The definition of insanity is repeating the same thing over and over and expecting a different result." It is time for change.

Now we are just waiting for the Swedish FDA to realize it. Perhaps it already has. They might have put together a twenty-year plan for a slow change of direction so that no one needs to lose his or her face. For example, in the fall of 2009, it eliminated the advice to eat bread with each meal. It's a tiny step in the right direction.

While our federal agencies slowly keep going and the food industry keeps resisting, we can ignore them. The madness ends now. It is time for the new world view to rise from the ruins of the old.

As you know, the new world view stems from millions of years of history. But we can start over in London in 1863. An overweight man was about to make a revolutionary discovery. It shows us the way forward.

II.
Forward

CHAPTER FOUR

A new but old solution

Of all the parasites that affect humanity I do not know of, nor can I imagine, any more distressing than that of obesity, and, having just emerged from a very long probation in this affliction, I am desirous of circulating my humble knowledge and experience for the benefit of my fellow man, with an earnest hope it may lead to the same comfort and happiness I now feel under the extraordinary change . . . which might almost be termed miraculous had it not been accomplished by the most simple common-sense means.

WILLIAM BANTING

William Banting didn't know it in 1863, but he was about to become famous in the entire Western world.

However, Banting did know that he had a problem. He was fat. Really fat. His funeral agency in London was successful and well off. But he had a difficult time being happy. Despite being short, he weighed 203 lbs (92 kg). He constantly failed any attempt to get thin. Instead he got heavier.

Obesity plagued him. His bloated belly had given him a painful umbilical hernia that had to be bandaged. His knees and joints ached and needed to be wrapped. Climbing flights of stairs was a challenge.

His descent was slow and backwards, and ascension left him short of breath and sweaty. He could barely tie his own shoelaces.

Being the heaviest man around created several issues. He was indeed perceived as having a very thick skin, but other people's gleeful laughter behind his back caused him to isolate himself more and more.

He had a difficult time understanding why he was obese. He led an active life and tried to eat reasonable portions. The rest of his family was thin. He repeatedly solicited doctors for help. Despite them being "neither few, nor of a less than stellar reputation," it led nowhere. Sometimes they told him that his obesity was incurable, sometimes he received new advice.

He tried them all. Smaller portions, more exercise, ocean air, Turkish baths, walks, laxatives, diuretics, horseback riding. Twenty or so attempts in just as many years didn't result in much positive effect on his weight. One time he starved himself so much that he was afflicted with abscesses and had to undergo surgery. To recuperate, he ate normally again after which he weighed more than ever.

One day everything changed. He had sought out an ear specialist, Doctor Harvey, for issues related to his hearing. Harvey had studied in Paris and had brought back a new idea. He suggested a new diet for Banting to try. As usual, Banting followed the new diet diligently. That day changed his life.

Suddenly he started losing weight. Not minor, temporary weight loss, but a constant loss, week after week. Despite eating until he was full, he lost about 2.2 lbs (1 kg) per week. Soon he had shed 46 lbs (21 kg). Banting was no longer a fat man. While the pounds disappeared, he regained his health. He was feeling the best he had felt since his youth.

After decades of hard work, he had found his solution and it wasn't even difficult. Quite the opposite, actually. He could not let other people unnecessarily suffer the same way he had. He had to tell them.

Banting wrote a pamphlet comprised of twenty or so pages about his story. He printed two thousand copies and handed them out for free. They quickly disappeared. And so did the following editions. Banting's book was a sensation. It was translated into all kinds of languages, even Swedish. His poplularity was such that the question, "Do you Bant?" referred to his method, and eventually to dieting in general.

Prominent doctors were skeptical of the diet. But thousands of handwritten thank-you notes from all corners of the world showed that it had had an effect on countless people. Banting continued to propagate for his diet for the rest of his life and managed to keep his new weight.

So what was the secret? What made Banting lose the extra pounds? He was to avoid sugar and starch. But he could eat himself full on other things. So Banting received the advice to avoid everything that was new in the human diet, that which we didn't eat during the first 364 days as hunter-gatherers. He was to refrain from sugar, bread, beer, and potatoes.

Despite that rule, every day was a party for Banting. Perhaps too festive. He could fill himself up on bacon for breakfast and fish and meat dishes with vegetables for lunch and dinner. Lunch and dinner were both accompanied by two glasses of wine. He also suggested a drink as a nightcap "if necessary." So there was a lot of alcohol, but he stayed away from the carbohydrates.

Banting explained the success in one way. He had been relentless in sticking to the recommendations he had received. From experience and after all the letters he had received, he was convinced of one thing. Those who only focused on portion sizes had made a huge mistake. The most important thing was not *quantity*, it was *quality*.

So what one eats was important to Banting, and how much was irrelevant. Recently, while we have become heavier, most people have believed the opposite to be true. That it is simply the quantity that counts: "Calories in and calories out." Now the theory starts to falter. Despite everything, Banting could have been correct. Like Martin Ingvar, neurology scientist and professor at the Karolinska Institutet, wrote in his book *Hjärnkoll på vikten* (2010): "It is *what* you eat that determines *how much* you eat."

Banting satisfied himself with calorie-rich food, downed with a calorie-rich wine, and still lost weight. How is that possible? The explanation is surprisingly simple, as we will see soon.

New York

Banting's story might sound too good to be true. If there had been a method to lose weight from eating good food, then why wouldn't everyone know about it today? Why is it that 150 years later, low-carb diets are still called a "fad" by antagonists?

There are several reasons, but only one that is important. If fat was dangerous, a low carbohydrate diet could not be good. We cannot see with open eyes until we let go of the fear of natural fat. During the last 150 years, numerous people have supported a low-carb diet as the most effective and simplest method of losing weight. The most famous of them was Robert Atkins, an American doctor.

In the beginning of the 1960s, Atkins had just opened his own practice in New York as a newly graduated heart specialist. He was thirty-three years old and the future should have looked bright. Instead he became distressed. "I looked forty-five years old," he later said in an interview. "I weighed 200 lbs (90 kg) and had three chins. I didn't get out of bed before nine and never saw patients before ten. I decided to go on a diet."

Atkins looked around for inspiration and decided on a plan from Dr. Alfred W. Pennington. Overweight subjects had lost weight by refraining from sugar and starch in their diets. Atkins hoped that the low-carbohydrate diet would help him lose a couple of pounds the first month. He quickly lost nine, then successively even more.

The young Atkins was hired by a company to help its employees lose weight. Out of sixty-five participants, he managed to get sixty-four down to average weight; the sixty-fifth person got halfway there. His reputation spread. He ended up on TV and in magazines. For some time, his diet was called "The Vogue Diet" after the magazine that had written about it. A publisher reached out to him and wanted to release a book to the general public. In September of 1972, the book *Dr. Atkins' Diet Revolution* was published. By Christmas, it had sold two hundred thousand copies, and six months later almost a million. As time passed, it exceeded ten million copies and became the best-selling diet book ever. Perhaps because the effect was so evident.

Atkins's low-carbohydrate method starts with a strict decrease of carbohydrate intake of twenty grams per day. Simplified, you eat meat, fish, eggs and natural fats such as butter and olive oil, and vegetables that grow above-ground (they contain fewer carbohydrates that those that grow below, like potatoes or root vegetables).

Carbohydrate-rich food should be completely avoided, such as sugar, bread, potatoes, pasta, and rice. After a couple of weeks or months on a strict low-carbohydrate diet, you can successively start increasing the amount of carbohydrates, depending on the effect on your weight.

Atkins followed the American dream and built a large enterprise around his diet. The commercialization wasn't all positive. They focused on replacement products for carbohydrate-rich food and candy. It is of course more difficult to make money off of real low-carbohydrate food like meat and fish. Under the brand Atkins Bars, they sold chocolate bars in which the sugar had been replaced by sugar alcohols.

Similar products are still sold as "low-carb" candy, even in Sweden. It is almost a scam, but perhaps it is ignorance. Half of the sugar alcohol is absorbed and becomes sugar inside the body, which the vendors knowingly ignore. The rest ferments due to intestinal bacteria and causes gas and diarrhea. Why not sometimes enjoy a small piece of dark chocolate instead?

Perhaps especially Americans want to believe that you can eat normally and still lose weight. It is only human to wish something so magical. And capitalism gives Atkins enthusiasts everything they dream of today: low-carb pasta, low-carb ice cream, low-carb bread, low-carb chips, low-carb cookies, diet soda with artificial sweeteners, etc.

I suggest you forget everything like that. In the United States I have met many low-carbohydrate enthusiasts who happily eat such products. If you ask me, that seems to be working out poorly. Many of those people have a hard time losing weight. Ironically, the man with the biggest weight problem had a company that sold low-carbohydrate products.

Instead you should keep a naturally low-carb diet, filled with meat, fish, butter, and vegetables. Food that has worked for us for millions of years. Not products that claim to be low-carb versions of the low-fat industrial food. To cut to the chase, it is the same crap with a different name.

Let's return to Robert Atkins. He advocated for his fatty low-carbohydrate diet while the fear of fat was at its strongest. Naturally, he was very controversial. I remember how one of my brother's very overweight friends tried Atkins in the middle of the 1990s. Dieting with beef and béarnaise sauce? During my medical studies, this sounded like madness to me, if not entirely life-threatening. But I remember that he became lean.

Atkins's enterprise grew into an empire rich enough to start supporting large and very expensive studies about low-carbohydrate diets. More and more started to lose weight using his method. The company's slogan eventually became: "Everybody knows someone who has lost weight with Atkins. Become that person."

One spring day in 2003, it all ended. Atkins, seventy-two years old, was on his way to work in New York after a blizzard. An icy spot ended his story. Atkins slipped, smashed his head against the pavement, and fell unconscious. His skull had cracked and the bleeding caused his brain to contract. He never woke up. After nine days in the ICU, he was dead.

As soon as Atkins was gone, the rumors started to spread. Atkins had "died from a heart attack and had been morbidly obese at the time of his death." That was not true. Atkins had lost the extra weight when going on a low-carbohydrate diet four decades ago. In photos taken later, you see an older gentleman with friendly eyes. He was of seemingly average weight if not on the thin side.

The rumors could not be stopped; they fit together too perfectly with the general fear of fat. Low-carbohydrate diets, which had been a growing trend in the United States, were starting to lose speed. Two years after his death, Atkins's business went bankrupt.

Njurunda, Sweden

Sweden has its own William Banting or Robert Atkins. Her name is Annika Dahlqvist, and she is just as controversial.

Annika Dahlqvist worked as a northern district doctor in 2004 when her life changed. As she would go on to write about in her books and talk about during hundreds of lectures, she had long had issues with her weight. She was constantly yo-yo dieting. As soon as she reached her ideal weight, she'd try to eat to satisfaction and she'd gain all the weight back.

From the beginning of the 1990s, she tried to solve the problem by keeping a low-fat diet. She was not going to eat fat anymore. From that day on, she says, "I lost all control over my weight." The hunger conquered her. Her daily dieting attempt was aborted when she found herself eating in the kitchen. She gained 44 lbs (20 kg).

She felt increasingly sicker. Her wrists and shoulders were swollen and ached. She injected her shoulders with cortisone every month, but the effects quickly dissipated. Attempts at losing weight with the help of long walks failed. Instead her knees started to ache. Her belly was rebelling with gas, bloating, and aches. Her muscles were stiff and achy. A fast work pace and dwindling energy led to exhaustion and sick leave. She didn't understand how you could become so "exhausted as a human" at the mere age of fifty-five.

In October 2004, her daughter returned home from medical school. Her daughter told her that she had done a group lab with different diets. Her group had tested a strict low-carb diet and she had lost 6.5 lbs (3 kg) in a week.

Annika Dahlqvist, who had tried virtually everything to no avail, immediately wanted to try it for herself. She hadn't lost 6 lbs (3 kg) in years. That winter she lost 2.2 lbs (1 kg) per week. She almost reached her ideal weight. Her hunger was gone.

After a couple of months she discovered that she had recovered from her ailments. Her shoulders and wrists no longer hurt and her stomach had become flat and calm. She considered it a miracle. She couldn't keep quiet. She gave the same advice to her patients, with excellent results. She started to write letters to editors, conducted interviews for magazines, and started a blog to spread the message.

Her message is that overweight people or diabetics should keep a LCHF diet. It stands for "Low Carb, High Fat," meaning fewer carbohydrates and a higher percentage of fat. In this book, I have referred to it as a low-carbohydrate diet for two reasons. Because it is clearer than an acronym, but also because similar food had a long history before it received the name LCHF in Sweden. But it is essentially the same. A significantly reduced intake of carbohydrates will always result in a higher percentage of energy from fat.

The publicity was not delayed. Annika Dahlqvist makes people react, often in a powerful way. With her relentlessly uncompromising style, she attracted a lot of media attention in tabloids and on TV. Soon, everyone had an opinion about her. For some, she is a heroine who states what everyone else keeps quiet about. Someone who has helped them to better health. For some, she is a red rag to a bull. To a dieting professor who has long advocated for a low-fat diet that made Dahlqvist both fat and sick, she is "a happy and fluffy enthusiast from the north."

Dahlqvist responds by calling dissidents part of "the establishment." If you are part of the establishment, it is implied that you are narrow-minded and denying reality, and if pushed to its extreme, also on the food and pharmaceutical industries' payroll. In other words, she is not afraid of conflict.

You can have reasonable doubts. Dahlqvist is more practical than theoretic. She has seen what works, but hasn't read all the studies. Her punchy but ill-conceived statements cause gaffes. Like Swedish tabloid *Aftonbladet*'s headlines in August of 2009: "THE FAT DOCTOR: MY DIET PROTECTS AGAINST THE SWINE FLU." That triggered a lot of criticism, even if the media provoked it. There was no evidence to support such a claim, and Dahlqvist soon retracted her statement.

Some can't handle spontaneous, categorical statements without scientific support, especially from doctors and those in the media. That includes many of my colleagues in the healthcare industry.

They get rashes from such things. Therefore, Dahlqvist's credibility is limited in those circles.

Despite the controversy, or thanks to them, Dalqvist makes a living from writing books (of the bestseller kind) and traversing the country with her lectures about LCHF. More and more try it and experience better health and weight, just like she did.

The modern Swedish version of a low-carb diet called LCHF, the one Dahlqvist made popular, is similar to the Atkins diet. But three differences have emerged.

There is no generally recognized limit for the percentage of carbohydrates, even though a maximum of 10 percent could be seen as a rough estimate.[1] It could be assumed that the fewer carbohydrates you eat, the more significant effect it will have on your health and weight.

So, you need to reduce the carbohydrate intake as much as you are comfortable with and continue as long as you need to. Some eat almost no carbohydrates at all, while others just reduce their intake.

The second difference is a strong focus on real food, cooked with natural ingredients (such as meat, butter, and vegetables), without unnecessary additives. Processed diet candy or pasta that claims to contain fewer carbohydrates is not recommended. No one is selling Dahlqvist chocolate.

Finally, we strive for a balance between omega-3 and omega-6 fat. Fatty fish and meat from animals that have grazed are good. However, people avoid an exaggerated intake of omega-6, contained within certain ingredients like cheap vegetable oils and margarines. Those kinds of things could be correlated with inflammatory diseases such as asthma.

Is a low-carbohydrate diet effective for weight loss and overall

---

1. Note that many, including myself, never weigh or count our food. If you stick to meat, fish, eggs, fatty sauces, some cheese, and a reasonable amount of above-ground vegetables, you would end up around with around 5 percent of carbohydrates. If you add additional vegetables, nuts and berries, cream, and some root vegetables, and a couple of diversions, you end up around 10 percent.

health, or is it a "fad diet" among many others? Today, science provides the answer. But first, let us note something funny about the three stories you just read.

The Swedish spark

When you read about Banting, Atkins, and Dahlqvist, the similarities are striking, right?

It's the same history, in nineteenth century England, in twentieth century United States, and in twenty-first century Sweden. Three successful people suffer from obesity and disease. After several failures, they try a low-carbohydrate diet and get healthy and thin. Then they teach the diet to other obese people who in turn spread the message. Eventually, all three became famous and highly controversial.

These are only three well-known cases. There are numerous similar stories from the past one hundred and fifty years. If fat makes you fat, or if the choice of food is irrelevant, then why do the same phenomena keep emerging? How can so many obese people, regardless of country and century, experience the same thing: a lifelong weight problem that ends when they stop eating sugar and starch?

Does science show something else? Does a low-carb diet work in practice, but not in theory? Do we have to choose between reality and the map? Or can they be married? I claim that we can do that today. In Sweden, we received help from an unexpected source.

In 2005, Annika Dahlqvist was reported to the National Board of Health and Welfare by two dietitians. Back then it was significantly more controversial to openly advise diabetics to eat fatty food. The dietitians claimed that it jeopardized patient safety. They wanted to stop Dahlqvist's advice. Ironically, their claim had the opposite effect. It became crucial for the following turn of events.

The National Board appointed an investigation that took more than two years. It carefully reviewed the science behind a low-carbohydrate diet. The conclusion came in January 2008. Annika Dahlqvist was cleared of all blame. The news struck like a bomb at every newspaper. In an infected media debate, the National Board of Health and Welfare had all of a sudden validated the controversial fat diet. The "extreme fad diet" that many people still viewed as life-threatening.

Soon, numerous professors who had previously been influential wrote to the Diatetic Association via a long and confuzed debate article in the *Journal of Physicians*. It urged the National Board to retract its approval of the low-carbohydrate diet that they thought was a mistake. The National Board stood by its decision, which caused an inflamed debate in the *Journal of Physicians* between the different camps. Just as in the general media, the debate is still ongoing.

The turn of events could hardly be more similar to a paradigm shift.

A growing number of enthusiasts have long advocated for it. But the ignited spark in Sweden was the National Board's validation of a low-carbohydrate diet in January 2009. So what exactly did it say?

The investigation's summary, what upset the masses, stated among many things: "In conclusion . . . the low-carbohydrate diet is said to be in compliance with beneficial clinical practices for weight reduction for the overweight and for type 2 diabetics on the basis that a number of studies have shown positive short-term effects and no harmful side effects have emerged."

That was dynamite. Low-carb diets had long been dismissed as a dangerous fad. Now, the National Board itself stated the opposite, that it had been scientifically proven to be effective and to not bring any known risks. The effect on the Swedish debate cannot be overstated. The balloon of rumors and hearsay suddenly deflated and the smoke screen evaporated. Now it is time to see what lies ahead.

The Revolution Gains Traction

Banting and Atkins made a mark in history. But their ideas never became mainstream back then. Countless practical experiences weren't enough to reshape our world view. The development today could lead farther. It could go all the way.

The difference from 1860 or 1960 is that we now have scientific evidence. Proof that fits with practical experiences, evolution, and history. The evidence that the National Board discussed in 2008 as well as even more up-to-date studies. Today the map and reality can become one. They can grow together in the new world view. Your health and your weight are connected.

Let's start with weight. Few things could more easily motivate people to change their lifestyles, since the effect can be seen and felt immediately. Improved health is a bonus, sometimes an unexpected one. Additionally, the new theory about weight regulation is truly fascinating. It not only works, but it's also beautiful in its logic.

Today, we need something new. As with similar areas, the old weight theory is eroding due to all the contradictions.

They say losing weight is easy: "Eat less, run more." Expend more calories than you eat. The problem? While more people are frenetically counting calories, we haven't become thinner; quite the opposite, actually. Instead we have become victims of an obesity epidemic. A couple of hundred years ago, we didn't know what a calorie was, and almost everyone was lean. Today, an increasing number of obese people know how many calories a medium-size order of fries contains, yet they are heavier than ever. Something isn't right.

Calorie-counting generally fails in scientific studies, and it rarely has a long-term effect on weight. Sure, you will lose a few pounds in the beginning, but within a couple of years you normally gain back just as much or more. Everyone's seen it: yo-yo dieting leads to obesity.

They repeat: "Eat less, run more." Everyone's heard it. If it is that easy, why do so many people fail? The unsought answer is always, "Fat people are . . ."

Fat people are lazy and gluttonous. I believe that is what most people feel deep down today. I used to think so myself back in the day, in the absence of a better explanation. I don't believe that anymore. Quite the opposite. It is not science; it is prejudice against obese people. It is old-fashioned moralization, suspiciously reminiscent of the Bible's deadly sins: sloth and gluttony.

The old world view gave us an obesity epidemic, sickening dieting methods, and prejudice. The new one leads to weight loss without hunger, plenty of food, and improved understanding.

It is time to change our approach. Let your weight show you the way.

CHAPTER FIVE

Weight loss without hunger

"It is just as stupid to think you become fat from fat to think that you become green from eating vegetables."

CHRISTER ENKVIST, CHIEF PHYSICIAN
DN *Debate 2004*

Chemical engineers connected with the large margarine enterprise Unilever are close to succeeding. They are experimenting with an edible jelly containing very few calories. Something that overweight people can eat instead of food or as an added element to ready-made food. The jelly is supposed to be soft when it is consumed and swell into a hard mass in the stomach. While it slowly breaks down, the appetite is repressed. Soon the only thing that will remain will be deciding which artificial flavoring should be added. They are hoping for a bestseller.

So the engineers are trying to create something that tastes all right, fills the stomach, suppresses hunger, and causes weight loss if necessary. That something already exists. It is called real food.

Today, no one recommends eating real food to lose weight. Instead they recommend low-fat products, powder, pills, or gastrointestinal surgery. What if all of this is based on a mistake? What if the whole billion-dollar industry is about to crash?

When you leave the fear of fat behind you, there is actually another alternative.

True but unusable

Do we gain weight because we eat more calories than we expend?

Thousands of obesity experts have for decades sworn that this is an indisputable natural law. Astonishingly enough, they are dead wrong. Sure, you have a surplus of calories if you gain weight. But there is a big hole in the logic of that sentence. The flaw is difficult to find, but once you do, it is evident. But first we need to understand more about how weight regulation works.

Blind faith in calorie-counting hides the problem. The mantra "calories in vs. calories out" is not a big help to overweight people. The calorie approach constitutes today's recommendation for weight loss: eat less and run more. The problem is that most people fail. Scientific studies and reality show a miserable long-term effect.

If you succeed in the long run with calorie dieting, congratulations. You must have an iron will or a lucky genetic makeup. Most people first lose weight. But then they gain all the weight back on, often more than they initially lost. They yo-yo diet their way to obesity. Few actually become lean. Even a fantastic human with personal chefs and trainers can end up in a vicious cycle of yo-yo dieting. Just look at Oprah.

With all imaginable advantages, how could you fail? Many experts have given up completely today, and assert that the only way to cure obesity is to surgically remove the stomach. It is difficult to envision a more complete failure for the calorie approach.

The problem is the oversimplified view of how your weight is regulated. The calorie fixation disregards the main question: *why?*

Why does every other Swede unwillingly eat too many calories? Why did the number of obese Americans quickly triple during the fear-of-fat era? Why did they see an epidemic of obesity, even amongst babies younger than six months? Do they have to run more? Why do you even want to eat more than you need to in the first place?

Understanding the cause can give you weight loss without hunger, also called the enjoyment method. What stands in its way is the fear of fat, that which Ancel Keys left us. You cannot recommend real food for weight-loss purposes if you think it is dangerous.

More carbohydrates, more insulin, more obesity. That correlation is the key to being overweight. Insulin stores fat in the fat cells and locks it down. If the insulin levels in the blood are high, your fat reserves are locked up and will happily increase in size. The volume of insulin in your blood can eventually determine your fat content.

It is easy to reconcile the effect of insulin with the talk about calories and weight. The easy way is to conclude that carbohydrates and insulin make you hungrier. Too much insulin makes you eat more than you need.

There is a more complicated and elegant way of seeing it. It might sound strange at first, but give it a shot. In the new world view, everything is turned upside down. Think about it: you don't gain weight because you eat too many calories. The correlation is there, but the cause is the opposite. You eat too many calories because you gain weight.

Let me explain.

Controlled by fat cells

Obesity is essentially an excessively large fat storage. This is caused by a malfunction of how the fat cells are regulated, which makes them grow too much.

We have seen the fat cells as a passive container where excess food is stored. That is incorrect; the fat cells are active. When they absorb nutrition, you gain fat weight. They extract the nutrition from the blood and you become hungrier and eat more. That is the effect of insulin.

Resisting such hunger is self-torture. You cannot win the battle against hunger in the long run; it always returns. But you don't have to resist it. There is a better way.

Perhaps you know someone who has lost weight with a low-carbohydrate diet. They always say the same thing. Suddenly the hunger and sugar cravings disappeared. Suddenly they felt satisfied longer. Now we can understand what happened: a morbidly high insulin level was normalized. The fat cells could release their repositories of nutrition, filling the blood with stored energy.

Growing vertically or horizontally

How can a hormone determine your fat weight? There is a good analogy. Charles, fifteen years of age, has a teenage body filled with growth hormone that makes him grow taller. He doesn't grow because he eats more. Quite the opposite, actually. He eats more because he is growing. If Charles got his act together and ate smaller portions, he would still keep growing.

Growth hormones makes Charles grow vertically. Insulin makes you grow horizontally. Both hormones activate cells and make them grow. The cells absorb nutrition from the blood, which results in hunger. A growing child needs extra food. An adult with a growing belly also needs extra food.

The correlation is inverted. You eat more than you expend because you gain weight. Because your fat cells are growing. If you can instead get your fat cells to shrink and fill your blood with nutrition, the opposite will happen. You will want to eat less than you expend. That causes weight loss without hunger.

Göran Adlén, a trend analyst dressed in black, coined the term *the enjoyment method*. He and half his family lost their overweight without hunger and with fewer carbohydrates. On New Year's Day 2009, Adlén appeared on *Good Morning Sweden* on Swedish National Television and foresaw that the country would have a massive breakthrough. He was right. Now Sweden is awakening, before any other country in the world.

Lean pigs and heavy humans

The enjoyment method has been around for hundreds of years. In 1825, Jean Anthelme Brillat-Savarin, a gifted chef and French national saint, published the book *The Physiology of Taste*, one of the world's most famous culinary books. In the book he describes what obese people eat. He had often heard them talk about it. He was sure of this. It was the same as back then: bread, rice, potatoes, cookies, and sweets.

It was unknown back then, but that food also transforms into sugar in the stomach. It raises the blood sugar level and insulin. The fat cells obey the insulin and store fat.

Brillat-Savarin noted that wild carnivorous animals never become obese. Not the wolf, jackal, lion, or the eagle. Predators barely eat carbohydrates at all. Their insulin stays low.

Those who have an overweight predator at home (dog, cat) today can control the content of their food. The fat domesticated dog doesn't eat meat like its wild forefathers. The fat dog eats carbohydrates instead because it is cheaper.

The biggest ingredient in pets' dry food is rice, corn, or grains: concentrated carbohydrates. That gives the dog high insulin levels and its fat cells swell. The cause of the dog's obesity could be the same as its owner's obesity. Neither of them eat what their bodies are designed for.

The bear is another great example. In the fall, it has to gain a significant amount of weight by adding a bunch of fat. It needs the fat reserve before it goes into hibernation during winter. So what does it eat? Blueberries. Tens of pounds of blueberries every day. Sugar.

Pigs are similar to humans. In the 1960s when they raised pigs for Christmas ham, the fat rim was supposed to be several inches thick. People wanted a fatty ham back then. The farmer raised fat pigs on potatoes and breadcrumbs. Now people want lean Christmas ham, and so the pigs are fed corn oil to become thin.

Ironically, the pigs back then became fat by eating low-fat food. But people who ate the fatty ham became thin. Today, the pigs become thin from the fatty food. But the people who eat the lean ham (with carbohydrates, bread, potatoes, beer, and Christmas candy) actually become heavier.

Bread and potatoes, food that we were recommended during the obesity epidemic, make pigs fat. It raises the insulin level and makes their fat cells absorb all the nutrition from the blood in order to grow. The pig becomes hungrier and eats more.

Humans work the same way. A surplus of carbohydrates, enough sugar, can make us fat like pigs.

Time to prove it

The new theory is logical. But it is more than a beautiful theory that fits with evolution. Today, there are scientific studies that have verified it in the most absolute terms. We are waiting for the answer. First, a quick recap of the background.

Since the 1980s and onwards, there have been no doubts. Fat made you fat, they said, without more proof than to show that vegetables make you green. Many believed that carbohydrates weren't even capable of causing weight gain, based on a misunderstanding. That era provided us with an obesity epidemic.

Modern science points in another direction. Those who previously recommended a low-fat diet have fully retreated. They are now backing a position that is almost indefensible: "All diets are equally good." As long as you count calories going in and out. *What* you eat doesn't matter. With that logic, ice cream, chocolate pastries, and soda are just as healthy for your weight as real food. Is that true?

In theory, it is enough to count calories. In reality, hunger is a factor. Real food keeps you satisfied longer. Candy and soda create an immediate craving. It is therefore not as easy to count calories as you may want to believe. Today, we can make science fit together better with common sense.

How do you prove which food causes the best weight loss? It is surprisingly difficult. You have to employ the sharpest tool science can provide. A fair comparative study between the alternatives.[2] Those take time and require many participants. They can cost hundreds of thousands or sometimes even millions of dollars. Still, twenty studies or so have been conducted during the twenty-first century, in which the two main alternatives have been compared. Today's low-fat, calorie-counting diet against the challenger, the low-carbohydrate diet without hunger.

For decades, dieters in the Western world have been recommended a low-fat diet for two reasons—fat was perceived as dangerous, and fat contains many calories per gram. There is no proof that that approach is beneficial for your weight. Finally, we have the test results for this method that fat people are using until many of them give up, and have their stomachs surgically reduced in pure frustration.

Thinner in America and Israel

What if the complete opposite is true? When the first eye-opening study was published in 2007, many shorter studies suggested that that might be the case. It was a study that was difficult to discard.

The study's main author was, ironically, a vegetarian. Christopher D. Gardner is a Stanford professor and had previously done research on soy, garlic, and vegetarian food. But when he presented his research at conferences, he received questions about other things. People wanted to know if the periodically trendy low-carbohydrate diets like Atkins actually worked, if they caused weight loss.

---

2. In order to impress doctors, you need randomized controlled studies (RCT). Obese volunteers are randomly divided into two groups that are charged with following two different diets. When a set amount of time has passed (like six months or two years) you see which group has lost the most weight, and whether or not the discrepancy is convincing or "statistically significant."

The randomization ensures that participants are divided fairly. If the participants get to choose a group, the groups may turn out too different. The most motivated participants might choose the same group and will therefore have an unfair advantage. The randomization ensures a fair study.

Gardner realized that, despite having been popular for a long time, there were no new studies that compared its long-term effects to those of other diets. He decided to answer the questions. After having collected $3 million of federal funds, he started a one-year study that is the largest to date.

He randomly divided 311 overweight people into four groups. One followed the Atkins diet, in other words, a strict low-carbohydrate diet that starts with twenty grams of carbohydrates per day. That equals about 4 percent. Sugar, bread, and potatoes should be avoided. Instead, the participants could stuff themselves with meat, fish, eggs, butter, fatty sauces, and above-ground vegetables.

The remaining three groups were recommended diets with a significantly higher proportion of carbohydrates, one of which equals what the Swedish USDA advises. All groups were treated to a couple of educational trainings with dieticians. They were then tracked and measured for a year to see what would happen.

The results were published in 2007 in the respected medical publication *Journal of the American Medical Association*. There was no doubt. The Atkins group statistically lost the most at all weigh-ins. But what surprised many people was the effect on the risk factors for heart disease.

The general consensus was that fat was bad for one's cholesterol, the main reason behind the fear of fat. But when this was tested, the group that kept a low-carbohydrate diet had *better* cholesterol levels and better blood pressure. Nothing seemed to have deteriorated.[3]

Dagens Nyheter used the headline FEWER CARBOHYDRATES IS THE BEST DIET, and started the article with: "Dieting women lose twice as much weight with the low-carb Atkins diet, compared to diets that limit the fat intake. This was demonstrated in the hitherto largest, longest, and most well-conducted study."

---

3. You can watch a 75-minute lecture and Q/A with Professor Gardner online. He talks about how low-carbohydrate diets recently have defeated the alternatives in increasingly larger studies, including his own, with the best impact on weight and risk factors. Search online for the lecture title: "The Battle of the Diets: Is Anyone Winning (at Losing)."

Was the study a one-time thing, a random coincidence?

In the summer of 2008, an even better study was published in one of the more renowned magazines for clinical research, *New England Journal of Medicine*. It remains the largest study that has ever been conducted on the topic of low-carbohydrate diets.

Led by the research director Iris Shai, 322 overweight people were randomly divided into three groups: Atkins, Mediterranean, or low-fat diet. The groups were tracked for two years. The participants worked in a nuclear power plant in the desert where they ate in cafeterias, which made it easy to give them the correct food.

Which diet group experienced the most effective weight loss? Again, Atkins. The worst? Again, low fat. Their cholesterol levels showed the same results. Atkins won again.

The media jumped on the results. Dagens Nyheter chose the headline FATTY FOOD MAKES YOU THINNER, and started the article with: "More fat and fewer carbohydrates is the best and healthiest way of losing weight. That conclusion, which goes against the recommendations from the USDA, came from the hitherto longest study about different diets."

Ironically, the newspaper illustrated the article with two women eating ice cream. Sugary ice cream is the opposite of a low-carbohydrate diet. A couple of days later, the media forgot everything that this and other studies had shown. The media has the memory of a goldfish when it comes to medical research. They start from scratch with every study.

The aforementioned examples are the two largest studies that have been conducted on strict low-carbohydrate and low-fat diets for the purpose of weight loss. Despite the fact that the low-carbohydrate group has eaten to satisfaction, they have won both times. Despite counting calories, the other group keeps losing.

The hunger caused by a low-fat, low-calorie diet takes its toll. Sugar and starch raise the insulin level and speed up the body's fat-storing processes. Trying to compensate with self-discipline is a constant uphill battle. That's why they lose.

Instead, if you could eat your fill of good food, you would have a downhill journey toward your dream weight. That's why the enjoyment method is a good fit.

10-0

There are more comparative studies of low-carbohydrate vs. low-fat/calorie diets. In total, there are at least twenty-one from the twenty-first century.

The results clearly point in one direction (see the chart on the next page). At best, the low-fat diets have managed to tie the game; that is to say, the results have not been statistically significant.

But time after time, the results have been unequivocal. In the one-star studies, low-carbohydrate diet has won ten times. The low-fat alternative has never won.

The score is 10-0. The winner is more formally confirmed in a systematic review of all the studies, a so-called meta-analysis. The latest one by the English researcher Michelle Hession et. al. was published in 2009. They added the results from thirteen randomized studies.

The results? Overall, the low-carbohydrate diet provided the largest weight loss, best blood lipids, best blood pressure, and fewer defections.

What about the low-fat diet? It performed the worst.

The map and reality

Why is it that even some professors still say that what you eat is irrelevant for your weight, when time after time they are scientifically proven wrong?

The easiest explanation is that they haven't had time to read the new research. Or they are so stuck in the old world view that they cannot accept anything else. Perhaps they trust their map too much to take notice of reality. Worst-case scenario, the explanation is something else.

*

Study	Participant	Months	Low Carb Group	Low Fat Group	Best weight loss
Brehm -03	53	6	4–12 %	55 %	**Low Carb**
Foster -03	63	12	4 % +	60 %	Low Carb
Samaha -03	132	6	6 %	55 %	**Low Carb**
Sondike -03	30	3	4–8 %	55 %	**Low Carb**
Aude -04	60	3	10–28 %	55 %	**Low Carb**
Volek -04	31	1,5	<10 %	60 %	**Low Carb**
Meckling -04	31	2,5	12 %	55 %	Low Carb
Yancy -04	120	6	4 % +	55 %	**Low Carb**
Stern -04	132	12	6 %	55 %	Low Carb
Nickols-R -05	28	1,5	4 % +	60 %	**Low Carb**
Dansinger -05	80	12	4–10 %	55 %	Low Fat
Truby -06	212	6	4 % +	55 %	Low Carb
Gardner -07	311	12	4–10 %	40–70 %	**Low Carb**
Ebbeling -07	73	18	40 %	55 %	Low Carb
Shai -08	213	24	4 %+	>50 %	**Low Carb**
Sacks -09	811	24	35–45 %	55–65 %	Low Carb
Brinkworth -09	118	12	4 %	46 %	Low Carb
Frisch -09	200	12	<40 %	>55 %	Low Carb
Yancy -10	146	11	4 % +	55 % (+ Xenical)	Low Carb
Foster -10	307	24	4 % +	55 %	Low Fat
Krebs -10	46	3	4 %	55 %	**Low Carb**
Meta analyses					
Nordmann -06	5 studies	6			**Low Carb**
Hession -09	13 studies	12			**Low Carb**

LC group: the column shows the percentage of carbohydrates in the low carbohydrate group's recommended diet
LF group: the column shows the percentage of carbohydrates in the low-fat group's recommended diet
Plus: the amount carbohydrates slightly increased with time
Best weight loss: bold with a subsequent star = statistically significant results
Greyish text: not statistically significant results

Perhaps it is too embarrassing to change your mind too quickly?

Their usual counterargument is to note that one of the studies above didn't show any clear difference and dismiss the rest. They say that the study shows that there is no difference and that "all diets are equally good."

That's incorrect. If you are not a statistician, the following analogy might explain why. A soccer team that repeatedly loses and never wins is of course worse than its opponents, not equally good.

For example, if the small island nation of Malta manages to tie a game against the Swedish national team, following a couple of losses, the teams are evidently not "equally good." If a sports journalist seriously wrote that, people would laugh. But when a professor uses the same logic about a weight-loss diet, he or she is taken seriously. Why?

Fortunately, some professors understand better today. One such professor is Martin Ingvar, professor of Karolinska Institutet. In his book *Hjärnkoll på vikten* (*An Iron Grip on Your Weight*), he summarizes the results of weight loss studies: "Thus, reducing the number of calories and fat produces worse results in the long run than strategies focused on carbohydrate intake."

The victory is unquestionable. The question is: *how* effective is the low-carbohydrate diet?

370 lbs (168 kg) lighter

Solveig recently ended up in *The Norwegian Journal of Medicine* after a miraculous transformation. She had always suffered from weight-related issues and had been in contact with the healthcare system since she was two. At sixteen, doctors measured her insulin levels, which were very elevated.

She was recommended the "Eatwell Plate model," low-fat food, dieting pills, and exercise. She became increasingly heavier. In the end she weighed 551 lbs (250 kg), despite regular exercise with a physiotherapist. She reported the treatment to the patient health insurance board since she grew more obese from following the advice. She was denied, with the motivation that the healthcare system had given her proper care.

Solveig sought out a new doctor when she was twenty-five years old and weighed 584 lbs (265kg). The new doctor took notice of her extremely high insulin levels. She was recommended a low-carbohydrate diet to reduce them and eliminate what was hindering her weight loss.

She reduced her carbohydrate intake to less than forty grams per day. During the first two weeks, she shed 37 lbs (17 kg). A couple of months later, she had lost an incredible 165 lbs (75 kg). Her weight loss slowed down to about 2.2 lbs (1 kg) per week. She was feeling healthy and was soon able to take small walks, which successively increased to about 6.2 miles (10 km) per day.

Two years later, she returned for a checkup. The doctor barely recognized her anymore. She weighed 214 lbs (97 kg). Her blood levels were normal, including her insulin level. She had lost 370 lbs (168 kg) by removing the barrier to weight loss (i.e., her insulin), caused by all of the carbohydrates that the health community had advised her to eat.[4]

Solveig may hold a speed record, but there are many other spectacular cases. Like the man from the north of Sweden who, in one year, shed 203 lbs (92 kg) to reach average weight. The method was the LCHF diet with a lot of wild game. Or Daniel Strandroth, a young man I know who lost 110 lbs (50 kg) and became thin in eight months.

Could this be normal?

---

4. The doctor who helped her and who published the case in the Norwegian journal is Sofie Hexeberg. She has conducted research and holds a PhD in nutrition.

   In 2010, Doctor Hexeberg published a book about how she successfully treats patients with a low-carbohydrate diet. Not just for weight loss but for diabetes, high blood pressure, and many other diseases. The book has been translated into Swedish and is called *Nytt live med riktig mat – Frisk med LCH*. [English: A new life with real food – healthy with LCHF] I highly recommend it.

On average: 26

The randomized study is the fairest way of determining a winner. But to know the true effects on the motivated participants, we need studies on people who have voluntarily chosen a low-carbohydrate diet.

At the research hospital in Kuwait (of all places), such a study was conducted. Sixty-six heavily overweight people were allotted about twenty grams of carbohydrates per day for year. However, they were allowed to eat as much as they wanted of everything else. The results?

From an average weight of 280 lbs (127 kg), they lost an average of 57 lbs (25.9 kg). Additionally, their cholesterol and blood sugar levels significantly improved. I used to think that sounded a little too good to be true. Now I have witnessed too many similar cases to have doubts. There are also several other impressive studies.

A Spanish study tested a strict low-carbohydrate diet with a Mediterranean twist for three months. The food was allowed to contain thirty grams of carbohydrates from vegetables per day. They ate a lot of fish, cooked with olive oil, and drank one or two glasses of wine per day. As per usual, they were allowed to eat until they were full. Forty healthy but fat people participated, and even after only three months the average weight loss was 31 lbs (14 kg). That is more than 2.2 lbs (1 kg) per week without hunger. Their blood pressure, cholesterol levels, and blood sugar improved significantly.

Thus, the Mediterranean diet can be combined with a low-carbohydrate diet. There is of course no scientific reason today why you should avoid saturated fat (like butter). But you can do it if you want, and still keep a low-carbohydrate diet. A low-carbohydrate diet with less saturated fat is not impossible; it is just unnecessary.

Let's return to the one-year study. Losing 57 lbs (26 kg) in a year is more than a pound per week. That seems to be the normal long-term average with a strict low-carbohydrate diet. It is also common to lose 4.4 to 6.6 lbs (2-3 kg) per week (or more) during the first few weeks, which is good for motivation.

Some shed weight more quickly, while others take a little longer. But if you can eat until you are full and still feel healthy, you are in less of a hurry. Additionally, with a slower pace, the skin has a chance to retract. When you approach a normal weight, weight loss slows down, until the weight is stabilized at a level where your body feels comfortable. Therefore, eating until you are full with food for which we are designed usually causes you to end up at a normal weight.

One question remains. What about exercise?

From coercion to a bonus

Caloric dieting isn't all about hunger. You also need to exercise, preferably hard and long. Just to burn off a cinnamon bun, you need to run 3.1 miles (5 km) or more. Exercise is good for your health and well-being but is overrated for weight loss. Studies show minimal or no weight loss without at least a one-hour hard workout each day. That sounds like self-torture if you are very overweight and lack energy. If you have other ailments, it can be impossible.

With a smarter dieting strategy, like that of William Banting, you don't need to work too hard. A low-carbohydrate diet allows you to eat until you are full, and if you don't want to exercise, you often still lose weight. Exercise is not coercion anymore, it is a bonus.

Surely exercise affects your weight. But reality is not as black or white like the drawing board theory claims about "calories in and out." Sure, you will lose weight from additional exercise *without extra food*. The problem is that exercising makes you hungrier. If you work outside in the forest, you are hungrier at night than if you have been stuck in an office all day.

If you replenish with a bottle of sugary "sports drink," you quickly negate the results from the workout. You expended sugar and replenished with more. That doesn't make you thinner or healthier. Like the triathlete Jonas Colting said: "Talk about digging a hole to put your ladder in so that you can clean the windows on the ground floor."[5]

If you want to exercise to lose fat weight, you should exercise under optimized fat-burning conditions. How do you do that? With a low level of insulin. How do you achieve that? By eating less sugar and starch. The more you exercise, the more insulin is needed to take care of the carbohydrates you eat (which equals easier weight loss), and the closer you get to average weight, the better it usually feels to work out. Welcome to a positive cycle.

Of course you get more energy to work out if you eat until you are full. Now you don't have to tax the body by exercising while hungry and tired. Instead you can exercise if and when you feel like it to feel good and become extra healthy. If you have a surplus of fat, it will burn off more quickly with increased exercise.[6] But it is no longer a coerced activity, it is only a bonus.

The fear of fat is becoming more and more disgusting.

"Calories in the air"

A doctor, a chief physician, produced a serious gaffe in a recent interview. The clinic no longer wanted to advise overweight people. According to the doctor, it was a waste of time because the effect was too poor. The journalist should have understood that you can't have "a bunch of fatties who refuse to lose weight and who occupy the dietitians' time."

---

5. Jonas Colting has long tried to highlight the issues with athletes' unnecessary gluttony of quickly digestible carbohydrates. In 2009 he wrote a recognized opinion piece about it in *Runner's World*. Search online for "The Carbohydrate Bluff" if you want to read it online.

Do you think you need to eat a lot of pasta and bread to have the energy to exercise? Tell that to Björn Ferry, who won an Olympic gold medal for Sweden in 2010 on a pure low-carbohydrate diet. Victories with a low-carbohydrate diet according to Ferry? Less body fat, more muscles. You can read more about it in his cookbook *Ferry Food* (2011).

6. In the future I am guessing most personal trainers will recommend their clients to combine their exercise with a low-carbohydrate diet for a reduced fat weight. It could provide them with an advantage. I already know a couple who have started, with great results.

Even for a doctor, it is frustrating to do your best and repeatedly fail. It is human to put the blame on someone else. But the main problem was not at all that fat people refuse to lose weight. The problem is that the healthcare community sticks to obsolete advice that performs the worst.

If you believe weight loss is simple, "eat less and run more," and the patients continue to be just as obese, what happens? Doesn't that risk *producing* prejudice? If it is that simple, the reason for obesity might just be poor character, gluttony, or laziness.

What the doctor didn't understand is that exacerbated hunger and energy deficiency isn't the *reason* behind obesity. They are the symptoms of a typical hormone disturbance, elevated insulin, which is the cause.

HIGH INSULIN

->

HUNGER, FATIGUE, WEIGHT GAIN

With a high insulin level that locks the nutrition in your fat storage, you become hungry, lack energy, and gain weight. Everything is interconnected. The healthcare community shouldn't expose their clients to prejudiced moralization that does no one any good. Instead, they should help treat the cause of the problem.

A while back, I was at a conference and listened to a lecture by a doctor. She was a specialist in clinical treatment of obesity with low-caloric recommendations. She didn't even seem to be admitting to herself that the treatment worked poorly. She seemed to take her frustration out on making ironic remarks about her patients' excuses: "there's something wrong with the scale," "there are calories in the air," and other derogatory jokes.

The old theory about weight regulation doesn't provide less obesity, but it generates prejudice. Even among doctors. Yet several of the conference attendees were offended, so surely there is hope.

The reason behind the failure is that a low-calorie diet often contains enough carbohydrates to elevate the insulin, trap the content of the fat cells, and produce hunger. The doctor's advice made it more difficult for her patients to lose weight, and then she scorned them for failing.

Just like with saturated fat, it is difficult and takes time to rethink. We have been convinced that fat is bad for our weight. In the absence of evidence, the same poor arguments are used.

Do you weigh your food?

Fat contains nine calories per gram, whereas carbohydrates and protein contain four. Therefore, they claim low-fat food produces weight loss. That is because if you eat the same amount of grams, low-fat food gives you fewer calories.

But who sits down at the dinner table with the intent of eating a specific amount of grams' worth of food, for example, 237 grams? Not me, and I'm guessing you don't either. The fear of "nine calories per gram" is thus a drawing board theory without a connection to reality.

If you have doubts, try out what makes you fuller in the long run: two hundred grams of cucumber or two hundred grams of meat fried in butter. What the food weighs is irrelevant. Your stomach isn't dictated by weight. You want to eat until you are full. That worked when we ate what we are designed to eat. If we return to that type of food, it works yet again.

Fat contains calories because fat is nutritious. If that was a problem, you would gain weight with an unlimited amount of a fatty, low-carbohydrate food. Studies prove the opposite is true. You more easily lose weight with this method than with other alternatives. Fat doesn't make you fat. Fat makes you full. Fill up on real food, and you can become thin without unnecessary counting or weighing.

It is time to stop following made-up rules. We don't have to count calories. Your body is designed to meticulously regulate your hunger, if you don't trick it with insulin-raising sugar and starch. Your lean ancestors didn't have calorie charts put away in their loincloths when they went hunting.

The alternative to real food is dieting candy, diarrhea pills, and brain surgery. See it for yourself.

Dieting with candy

Why do pharmacies recommend chocolate candy to obese people? Two chocolate pieces wrapped in plastic foil is suggested as a meal replacement. That's because they only amount to 240 calories.

The nutrition labels state: sugar, lactose, fructose syrup, fructose, sugar again, and glucose syrup. Six different versions of sugar. Even official dietary advice recommends a maximum of 10 percent of energy from sugar. That is a lot, many more times the amount that our ancestors ever consumed. In this piece of chocolate, which obese people are advised to eat instead of food, is not 10 percent, or even 20 percent. A staggering 34 percent of calories comes from pure sugar. The chocolate piece looks like candy, tastes like candy, and is candy.

How can it be good for your health to switch out food for candy? In theory, your weight goes down if the candy provides a caloric deficit. But that assumes an inhuman willpower. You will not feel full from a piece of chocolate for dinner. Why does a pharmacy facilitate such cynical fraud? Probably because they don't understand better. Their press reps explain that they sell chocolate candy as dieting aids because the customers demand it. I wonder what will be next. Cigarettes? Cocaine? Prostitutes?

The market is filled with companies that sell candy as "dieting aids" to overweight people. Herbalife, Optifast, Slimfast, and others, for example. After all, it is very lucrative. Sugar is cheap and can be sold expensively with shameless marketing.

But it is not only Swedish pharmacies that have let the candy in. I recently visited the American obesity doctors' annual congress in Seattle. Numerous candy providers showed off their products. They wanted doctors to recommend their specific calorie-counting chocolates, chocolate cereals, cookies, desserts, juices, and chips to their overweight patients. One even had a product for obese patients that don't like calcium pills to fight osteoporosis. Instead he sold chocolate and lemon muffins with added lime.

Ironically, the calorie-fixated doctors saw obesity as a chronic disease. Obesity "could not be cured." Instead, patients had to be treated for the rest of their lives with numerous preventative medications for risk factors. Perhaps soon all medications can be added to lemon muffins?

Many intelligent people have fallen for the failed calorie theory. Sweden's most famous dieting professors used to say that it would have been equally effective to diet with ice cream. That's how drawing board dieting works. It revolves around calorie counting rather than real food or common sense.

Even if in reality you don't get any leaner with ice cream, it works perfectly in theory.

The dream of the magic pill

For a long time, all hope was put toward a magic pill that would solve the problem. With that pill you'd be able to eat the same junk food and still get lean. Eat the cake and have it, too.

Today this looks more and more like a fantasy. Recently we had three options. The drug Reductil caused heart attacks, so it was forbidden. Alternative two, Acomplia, affects the brain and reduces your desire to eat. Unfortunately it reduced the desire for anything. For some, the fun was over. Many people got depressed, some committed suicide, and Acomplia was eventually forbidden as well.

What remains is Xenical, which is sold over the counter and in a lower dose under the name Alli. It provides a couple of pounds of weight loss by hindering the intestinal absorption of fat. The problem is that the fat you consume exits the other way instead. Common side effects according to the Swedish national formulary of drugs include: gas with possible oily excretion, sudden feces, fatty or oil feces, soft feces, stomach ache, as well as fecal incontinence. Finally, unsurprisingly: worry.

If you ask me, Xenical/Alli is pretty worthless. That pill cannot be combined with real food unless you want to spend the rest of your life in the bathroom. It can only be consumed with low-fat products. I never recommend it to my patients.

Transforming your body instead of your diet

If calorie-counting works poorly, pills work worse, and dieting candy works the worst, then shouldn't people have given up on the old calorie theory by now? Wrong. One last solution remains.

Few manage to starve themselves through strict self-discipline and ignoring hunger for the rest of their lives. Would you? But if the body doesn't obey, it can be coerced. You can surgically remove your stomach. It is effective, for good and bad reasons.

The most common surgery is called gastric bypass. The surgeon removes the stomach and the upper part of the small intestine. Only a little pocket of the stomach remains. Then you can only eat a couple of bites and drink a few sips before you become full. If you eat more, you risk vomiting. The fact that a piece of your intestine has been disabled impairs the absorption of the nutrition from the little food you are able to take in.

Unsurprisingly, most people shed a lot of weight after such a surgery, at least in the short run. They starve themselves whether they like it or not. Their body weight can drop several pounds a week. That is the big advantage.

Of course the surgery isn't risk-free. Serious complications and death can occur. The latter is rare, but I have personally met a woman who, a month later, died on the operating table. Her aorta had ruptured.

There are at least three common problems. The skin doesn't have enough time to retract as quickly as the weight drops. There is often a lot of excess skin that could require several plastic surgeries funded from your pocket, if you want to look better naked.

The second problem is that you risk nutritional deficiency for the rest of your life after disabling the stomach. The lack of vitamin B can cause dizziness and, worst-case scenario, also brain damage[7]; calcium deficiency can cause osteoporosis; and iron deficiency can cause anemia. It is especially worrisome when teens and future mothers undergo the surgery.

Finally, it is common to gain the weight back, especially if you keep eating the same type of food. After a year, the stomach has expanded, you can eat larger portions again, and the weight starts to go up. It is not uncommon to end up at a pre-surgery weight level.

Despite the disadvantages, obesity surgeries are becoming increasingly ubiquitous. A couple of years ago, barely anyone underwent them. Today, seven thousand Swedes annually have the surgery. There are more than a million obese Swedes, so in the future the surgery might become a routine treatment. Perhaps you need to disable your stomach.

How clear can it be? We don't live the way our bodies are designed. When we don't see through the mistake that makes us *want* to eat, we are forced to operate on our bodies so that we no longer can.

Food should be adjusted to our bodies. Not the other way around.

---

7. The medical journal recently wrote about a twenty-three-year-old woman who, after her gastric bypass, despite vitamins, suffered from severe B-vitamin deficiency. Her brain stopped functioning properly. The dizziness got worse and she experienced double vision. After three weeks in the hospital with large doses of vitamins straight into her bloodstream, she returned home. A couple of months later she still had a difficult time reading or watching TV and didn't want to risk driving a car.

A couple of hundred similar cases have been reported in the United States, of which half fully recovered. The memory and walking issues often remained.

Good advice before the knife

Before you decide on a risky surgery, the healthcare community should provide effective advice about natural weight loss, based on science and experience. That happens too seldom today. Unfortunately, healthcare professionals still believe in the dangers of fat.

Obese patients often receive recommendations that perform the worst in studies. Advice that makes it more difficult for them to lose weight. Those who fail are offered obesity surgery. Isn't that sick?

Ironically, many people who undergo gastric bypass surgery are worried that low-carbohydrate diets contain a high percentage of fat. But after the obesity surgery, the body is fueled by at least the same amount of fat. When you barely eat anything, the energy comes from the fat storage. Therefore, the body runs on fat-burning.

The positive effect of an obesity surgery is thus similar to the effects of a low-carbohydrate diet. In both cases, the carbohydrate intake is minimized, the insulin drops, and the body releases its fat-deposits.

You don't have to remove your stomach to eat a low-carbohydrate diet. Why not try that first? Doctors have an old saying: uncut is the best.

Next: the Cuckoo's Nest

It is about to get worse. How about some brain surgery à la the Cuckoo's Nest?

I am not kidding. In several countries, including Denmark, they are experimenting with placing electrodes in the brain. That is supposed to affect the appetite center and reduce your hunger. That is considered the next step after a failed gastric bypass surgery.

Carol Poe, sixty, was among the first women to undergo the surgery. She had tried every diet, undergone a gastric bypass surgery, and was still fat. She let herself be filmed for TV.

The inside of the brain has no feeling, so she is awake throughout the procedure. Thin needles are inserted into her brain carrying an electric current. She reports how it feels to guide the surgeon toward the appetite center. When the needles eventually hit the right spot, she craves her favorite drink, Pepsi.

Later, with the brain electrodes in place and the grey, stubby hair beginning to grow back, Carol welcomes the journalists into her home. She has lost 3 lbs, she says, and her cravings have been reduced. She shows her refrigerator. Only one of the Pepsi drinks has been opened. With a fascinated expression, she says that she opened it three days ago and has only drunk a couple of glasses. Before the brain surgery, she had a bottle a day, about two liters of sugar solution. Almost half a pound's worth of sugar each day. Enough to make anyone fat.

So we are surgically removing stomachs and undergoing brain surgery instead of quitting drinking soda. Our bodies are operated on to be able to take industrial food. Real food is switched out for chocolate candy from the pharmacies. Where is it going to end?

Away from the dead end

Hopefully it ends here. The fear of fat and calories is eroding in light of new science and common sense. Large studies show that fat and calorie restriction is the worst method for controlling your weight. Extreme and desperate solutions are thriving, but they will not stick around for long.[8]

The new view on weight control is ready to take over. It doesn't require hunger, pills, or experimental surgery. All you need to do is go back to eating real food again, like our ancestors did: meat, fish, vegetables, and eggs.

---

8. What is the issue with us "gaining weight because we consume more calories than we expend"? The issue is the word "because." It doesn't belong here. Of course you have gained more calories than you have spent if you gain weight. But that doesn't say anything about the cause or why you did it.

If you only hear discussion about calories, you might want to ask, "What is the reason for it?" until you hear a good answer. Something more thought through than moralization about the character of overweight people, almost half of the Swedish population. If you don't receive a proper answer, you can give the person this book.

Real food decreases insulin levels. For overweight people, the flow is reversed. The fat cells shrink and release nutrition into the blood. You feel fuller and get more energy to move: "calories in" decrease, "calories out" increase. You avoid hunger and fatigue and don't have to work out more than you are comfortable with. The enjoyment method enables you to work with your body in a smart way.

Instead of counting calories, you can listen to your body and feed it what it needs. You don't have to count calories more than you have to count the number of breaths you take. The body handles that for you, unless you trick it with food for which we are not designed.

It isn't just your weight that improves, but also the risk factors for heart disease. Your blood pressure, blood sugar, and cholesterol improve. It is not about weight, but overall health. If you doubt it, try it for yourself. It is simple, safe, and the food can be both inexpensive and tasty. In the end of the book there is a beginner's guide with practical advice.

Sweden could be a pioneer in this area as well. It is the country that is seeing the quickest return of real food, the first country to become thin and healthy again, the country that is paving the way. It is a place where people eat plenty of tasty food and get the desire and energy to move as a bonus.

The problem is concentrated sugar and starch, the new food that didn't exist before, that for which we are not designed. The kind of food that raises the blood sugar and insulin, the body's fat-storing hormone, and elevated insulin levels cause the fat cells to absorb nutrition and grow, which makes you heavier. It makes you hungrier and prompts you to consume more calories. A growing belly inevitably makes you hungrier for the same reason a teenager with a growing body is hungrier.

Calorie fundamentalists claim that food choice doesn't matter, but rather that "it is all about calories." They seriously think candy can give you a better weight than real food. As previously discussed, that idea works in theory, but not in reality. In theory, you can disregard hunger, but in reality, it is always a factor. Denying basic biological urges will hardly lead to anything good. Ignoring hunger could risk causing eating disorders like bulimia.

Yesterday's failed calorie theory advises us to eat the food that we use to fatten animals, and then recommend the solution of surgically removing our stomachs. That is, of course, insane.

But you haven't heard it all yet. Being overweight is only an early symptom of the Western disease. Eventually the long-term consequences of obesity kick in. When your blood becomes too full of glucose, you really have a problem.

CHAPTER SIX

Diabetes and the end of the madness

I have a difficult time understanding why the Swedish USDA recommends a low-fat diet and that this is then recommended to diabetics. . . All logic goes against it . . .

FREDRIK NYSTRÖM
Professor of internal medicine, Linköping University Hospital

A conversation in the dairy aisle with a stranger recently changed Kennet Jacobssons's life.

Kennet was forty-three years old when he was diagnosed with type 2 diabetes in the beginning of the 1990s. He was initially treated with pills, but soon he required insulin injections, in increasingly large doses, to regulate his blood sugar—the continuous deterioration that diabetics usually go through.

He soon suffered from major complications. His arteries were clogging up. He had a heart attack, then another one, and in the end he had had seven. In 2005 they opened up his chest and connected new arteries to his heart.

The incision wound got infected and he had to undergo a second surgery. He had to spend ten days with an open chest while they removed the bacteria. Broken ribs, morphine, and infections made him feel worse. In the end, he required twelve different types of medicine. Severe aches in his shoulders required cortisone injections. His future looked bleak.

On Sunday, August 2, 2009, Kennet was standing in the dairy aisle and started "talking about butter" with a stranger. The man told him that he and his wife had kept a LCHF diet for two years, in other words a strict low-carbohydrate diet. She had reversed her diabetes and lost 79 lbs (36 kg), and he himself had lost 18 lbs (8 kg) and felt excellent.

Kennet became curious. He got the link to the low-carb online forum *kolhydrater.ifokus.se* and started reading. He tried it out immediately. A week later, he had reduced his insulin dose from sixty-six to ten units per day. Yet his blood sugar level was better than before. After two weeks he had lost 18 (8 kg) out of his 251 lbs (114 kg), and his shoulder pain was gone. He was able to stretch his arms over his head, which had previously been impossible. Overall he felt much better.

A couple of months later, the number on the scale only had two digits and a pair of pants he hadn't fit into for ten years suddenly fit. Christmas and its associated fatty food provided an additional couple of pounds of weight loss. By the summer he had lost over 55 lbs (25 kg). He no longer needed the insulin or the medicine for heartburn and aches. His blood pressure was 130/80 without treatment. After a visit to the doctor's office in April, he packed a bag of leftover medicine to return to the pharmacy. From twelve, he was down to two medications.

Kennet is an exception—he managed to break the deterioration that usually comes with the disease. The day he stopped trying to follow the low-fat dietary recommendations and started to eat the opposite way, everything changed for him. When he stopped eating food to which human genes haven't had time to adjust, he became healthier and thinner. His sugar disease disappeared. The story is remarkable. Or is it?

A sneaky disease

Something is wrong. Many, if not most, people suffer from some kind of symptom of the Western disease. These consequences can kill us prematurely. The most extreme version of the disease causes what we call type 2 diabetes.

It is actually called diabetes mellitus, which means "sweet urine." That is because if the blood sugar is high enough, it leaks into the urine. The name provides a clue to how doctors used to diagnose the disease back in the day. Lucky for them, it used to be a rare disease.

The elevated blood sugar in diabetes damages the small blood vessels in the body. At its extreme, it corrodes the vessels. Poorly controlled diabetes slowly breaks down the organs in your body.

The kidneys stop working. Reduced blood flow in your feet can make them cold, reduce their sensitivity, and give way to infected lesions that don't heal. Eventually the toes might have to be amputated, then the feet, or more. Men often lose their sexual potency. The brain may be damaged and cause premature dementia. Eventually you risk going blind. The list continues.

Fortunately, it seems like the consequences of diabetes can be avoided. If you can normalize your blood sugar and insulin, the deterioration can be slowed down or stopped.

There are two main forms of diabetes. Type 1 diabetes used to be called juvenile diabetes. It is the rarest form today, but the easiest to understand. Your insulin-producing cells die, often at a young age. The insulin deficiency keeps your body from using the blood sugar and you quickly lose weight. It used to be a rapidly fatal disease. Type 1 was treated throughout life with meticulously measured insulin injections. You add what the body is lacking, and the problem is at best under control.

Type 2 diabetes used to be called adult-onset diabetes, since it almost only affected old people. However, its frequency has increased simultaneously with the obesity epidemic, and today even middle-aged and younger people are affected. Today in the United States certain obese children get adult-onset diabetes before their tenth birthday. No one knows what will happen to them in the long run.

Type 2 is by far the most common form of diabetes. It predominantly affects people with abdominal obesity. How do you know if you are sick? Perhaps you don't. The symptoms are unclear and can be missed for years, despite the fact that your body is undergoing repercussions. Sugar leakage into the urine produces larger urine quantities and increased thirst. Fatigue is also common. The diagnosis can be confirmed if a blood sample shows elevated blood sugar.

Type 2 diabetes means you have a bad case of the Western disease.

A health catastrophe

More people have developed type 2 diabetes since we became scared of fat. Here is the number of diabetics in the world, according to the WHO and the International Diabetes Federation, IDF:

1985: 30 million
1995: 135 million
2010: 285 million
2030: 438 million (prognosis)

The president of IDF, Jean Calude Mbanya, recently commented: "The epidemic is out of control. We are losing ground in the battle for slowing down the diabetes development." No one is discussing turning the development around, since they haven't even been able to slow it down. Swedes are hardly an exception. Healthcare professionals now meet type 2 diabetic patients daily. You probably know a few diabetics yourself. What is the reason behind the disaster?

The conventional explanation is familiar: people eat too much and run too little. Too much calorie-rich food makes them fat, in turn increasing the risk of diabetes. Is that true, or simply a moralizing whitewash?

Today, type 2 diabetes is considered a chronic disease that normally deteriorates every year. Patients receive the advice to eat less, especially less fat and saturated fat. This essentially means they need to eat more carbohydrates to feel full. With an increasing number of medications, they then try to control the blood sugar and other risk factors. The increasingly glucose-heavy blood that follows and its oftentimes disabling side effects is called the normal progression. We doctors aren't making patients healthier. We are administrating the decay, and the end is rarely beautiful.

But the situation isn't entirely hopeless.

Lard and cucumber

A historical perspective sheds light on today's diabetes treatment. In the beginning of the twentieth century, prior to modern medicine and insulin injections that could hide the problem, diabetes was treated differently. Without blood sugar-lowering medications, only one thing remained—avoiding the food that raised it in the first place.

Erik Ask-Upmark, a legendary professor of medicine in Uppsala, told his class how as a medical student, he experienced the era prior to insulin treatment. Sick diabetics received "every other day lard and cucumber, every other day cucumber and lard," so an extremely low amount of carbohydrates.

In 1923, Professor Karl Petrén, from Lund University in Sweden, published a book of almost a thousand pages about diabetes. His recommended diet had been popular for a long time. It was a low-carbohydrate diet, with unlimited amounts of pork, butter, and cabbage. Alcohol in the form of Bordeaux wine and hard liquor was also advised.[9]

Even during WWII, Swedish diabetics received extra cream, pork, or butter—if they didn't utilize their sugar ration.

---

9. Interestingly, red wine and hard liquor are the types of alcohol that contain the fewest carbohydrates. Useful knowledge even today for those who want to lose weight or improve their blood sugar level.

To avoid sweet drinks, you can order a vodka soda with lime instead, or a scotch. Beer is worse. It contains a lot of malt sugar, perhaps the reason behind the phenomenon "beer belly."

So, successful treatments prior to the era of insulin reduced the carbohydrates. The cookbook *Diabetic Cookery* from 1917 can be read online for free (find it online). It recommends fat- and protein-rich food. Page twelve lists food that "because of its high nutritional value is especially valuable," such as meat, fish, eggs, cheese, and butter.

On page thirteen, you can read about the types of food diabetics *shouldn't* eat. It includes sugar- and starch-rich food such as bread, rice, pasta, and root vegetables. The headline is telling: "Food strictly forbidden."

In 1917, bread, potatoes, pasta, and rice were absolutely forbidden for diabetics. Today the opposite is true: diabetics are recommended to eat predominantly from those food groups. In other words, they are advised to eat starch, which breaks down the glucose in the stomach and is absorbed as blood sugar. Diabetics are thus advised to eat blood sugar-raising food. That sounds crazy. What is the reason behind it?

The main reason for today's dietary advice is the fear of fat. Diabetics have an increased risk of heart disease. Since we used to believe fat was dangerous for the heart, they guessed that it was extra important for diabetics to avoid fat. Instead they needed to eat blood sugar-raising carbohydrates. They had to eat something. They tried to compensate for the blood sugar rush with more medication.

Now, when fat has been proven to be safe, the foundation for today's strange dietary advice is eroding. Does it have any evidence?

Proof level C

Evidence-based medicine is an attempt to make the healthcare community stick to treatments for which there exist evidence. "Evidence" means proof. The strength of the evidence is graded in different ways. One way is to let grade A equal the strongest and C the weakest type of evidence. In 2004, a European council of experts published a set of dietary advice for diabetics to which many refer. They advise diabetics to avoid fat. This piece of advice was attributed evidence grade C.

The following comments were made about the council's advice:

The recommendations about fat intake for diabetics is predominantly based on studies on non-diabetics.

It sounds like a joke, but it isn't.

Then there is the advice that diabetics should consume a lot of carbohydrates, upward of 60 energy percent. That, too, has the evidence grade like the advice about fat.

Evidence grade c is the weakest form of evidence. With certain studies you received grade a, good evidence. With more ambiguous and unsure studies that still support the advice, you received grade b, mediocre evidence.

Grade c means that there is no scientific study that supports the theory. Instead it relies on opinions from respected authorities. The dietary advice about how many carbohydrates diabetics ought to eat is thus based on people who should know, who instead *think* that carbohydrates are good for diabetics.

It doesn't help that the main author of these European dietary recommendations has worked as a consultant in the sugar industry. Regardless of what you make of that detail, there exists no evidence for the blood sugar-raising advice that diabetics have received for decades. Does that sound strange?

SBU, the Swedish government's council for medical evaluation, recently evaluated the scientific support for the Swedish dietary advice to diabetics. The report was published in the spring of 2010. We will soon get into the details of that interesting story. But the conclusion about today's low-fat dietary advice for diabetics is telling. The recommendations have "no scientific support."

You don't have to read a single study to prove something completely different yourself.

Sugar shock

How should you know what to believe? Try it yourself. Test your blood sugar before and after two meals. I will provide a funny example. I am not a diabetic, but the difference is still shockingly large. If I had been a diabetic, it would have been even bigger.

The worst lunch I had eaten in years was ironically served at the weeklong World Obesity Conference in Stockholm 2010. For lunch, the attendees were offered a dry sandwich, sweetened yogurt, an apple, and a chocolate bar (Dajm or Bounty). There was no alternative.

The food was almost all pure sugar or starch[10], new Western-food that raises the level of fat-storing insulin. But what does it do to your blood sugar? I sacrificed myself for science and tested it. I then compared it to a real meal. Meat, broccoli, and mushroom sauce with cream; real food. I had water with both meals.

This is what my blood sugar looked like after the two meals:

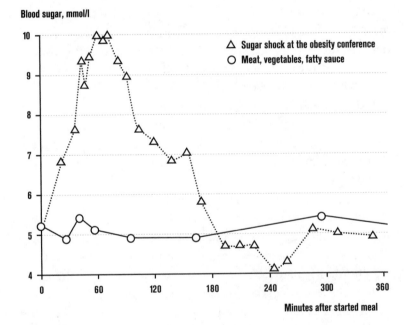

10. Sure, there were wild apples back in the day. But they weren't cultivated to be large and sweet, and didn't exist all year round, only seasonally. If you want to lose the weight that can cause diabetes, I suggest approaching sugary fruit as natural candy. Eat it occasionally because it is tasty. Fruit doesn't contain anything you need. You can easily get vitamin c from vegetables.

With real food, my blood sugar remained stable and unchanged. The body can easily handle the small amounts of carbohydrates.

As for the conference food, the sugar and starch, my blood sugar was spiking before I had even finished the meal. Half an hour later, it peaked at 9.9 mmol/l before it began to sink.

Note that the conference lunch caused the blood sugar to propel down after a couple of hours and become lower than before. That's when I was craving coffee and cake. With sugar and starchy food, you often get hungry more rapidly and risk eating more than you need, which causes weight gain.

This curve still counts as healthy. For someone with type 2 diabetes, the results probably would have been much worse.[11]

It seems evident which type of food is the best for diabetics that easily get high blood sugar. But you don't have to take my word for it. Plenty of studies show similar results. But you don't have to care about those either. The test is easy and free to try for yourself, and then you will know.[12]

Carbohydrates raise the blood sugar, which is why diabetics should avoid them. It is really that simple. Today's fat-resenting dietary advice for diabetics has zero scientific support.

Today's advice is showing to have unexpected repercussions.

Dangerous medication

Today's carbohydrate-rich dietary advice increases the need for blood sugar-reducing medication. These medications have in many cases

---

11. Two hours after you have consumed 75 grams worth of glucose (a test meal), the blood sugar is normally up to 8.7 mmol/L. Impaired glucose tolerance: 8.7–12.1. Diabetes: over 12.1. I was at 7 mmol/l, two hours after the horror food, so my blood sugar is normal.

Want to read more about blood sugar? See kostkotorn.se/diabetes

12. Search online for "blood sugar meter free" and you can get a free meter mailed to your house along with a couple of test sticks. You can purchase more sticks at a pharmacy for less than a dollar.

Test your blood sugar before and one hour after two meals. One meal with a lot of sugar/starch, like potatoes or whole-grain bread. One without, like meat, butter, and vegetables. Be amazed by the difference.

not been proven to be good for the health of type 2 diabetics.[13] It has not been proven that they live longer or become healthier from things such as insulin, beyond the elevated levels their blood already contains.

With the enormous ACCORD study in the United States and Canada, they wanted to finally show that an intensive medication regimen for blood sugar saves type 2 diabetics patients from heart disease. Over ten thousand diabetics were randomly divided into intensive treatment or control (non-intensive treatment). In the intensive group, they reduced the blood sugar with the help of insulin and often two to three additional blood sugar-lowering medications per day.

The bomb dropped in February of 2008. After the study had been ongoing for two years, it had to be prematurely shut down due to safety issues. The intensely treated participants didn't become healthier; quite the opposite. Many had gained over 22 pounds (10 kg) and suffered from severe blood sugar drops due to the medications. But that wasn't the worst thing. The intensely treated participants didn't even live longer. Rather, they died more quickly. The modern medication killed more diabetics than if they had kept their blood sugar levels elevated.

The ACCORD study demonstrates the intellectual meltdown behind modern treatment of type 2 diabetes. The unnecessary fear of fat led to advice about eating blood sugar-raising carbohydrates instead. Medication that would typically normalize elevated blood sugar has now been found to be life-threatening.

Doctors and other healthcare professionals obviously want what is best for their patients. But sometimes patients are unintentionally harmed by lack of knowledge. For example, phlebotomy was the most common treatment for most diseases long into the nineteenth century. It then turned out to be useless and oftentimes dangerous. Just like today's low-fat dietary advice.

---

13. The only exception is the first example, the pill treatment with Metformin, which has proven to be effective. It is easy to combine a low-carbohydrate diet with Metformin if more effect on the blood sugar is needed.

  If necessary, the next wise step could be so-called GLP-1 medication in injection form, like Byzetta and Victoza. It generates weight loss, not the opposite, like insulin.

We need something better. Something that doesn't make type 2 diabetics sicker, but rather healthier. A treatment that doesn't kill them prematurely.

Karlshamn and the world

Jörgen Vesti Nielsen worked as a chief physician at the medical clinic in Karlshamn when he saw the impossible. He met a patient who had lost 44 lbs (20 kg) and eliminated his diabetes by eating more fat. The patient had followed the Atkins diet.

Nielsen realized it might not be impossible after all. The patient had simultaneously eaten fewer carbohydrates. Nielsen started studying and found that studies actually showed better weight loss with fewer carbohydrates. But he couldn't find any studies on diabetics and low-carbohydrate diets. So he started his own.

The study was not one of those gigantic studies that pharmaceutical companies commission, with thousands of patients that are required to prove more subtle health effects. Nielsen's study was small. Therefore it would only prove obvious health effects. Sixteen diabetics were recruited and recommended a moderately strict low-carbohydrate diet (20 percent carbohydrates), and fifteen were assigned to the control group that followed the low-fat Eatwell Plate model (55-60 percent carbohydrates).

After six months, the difference between the groups was incredible. Those who kept a low-fat diet experienced no significant changes, probably because they had eaten the same way before, while they got sick. Those who were advised the low-carbohydrate diet had lost a lot of weight, on average over 24 lbs (11 kg). Additionally, their blood sugar had improved significantly, despite them being able to reduce their medication (three were able to quit insulin completely), and their good cholesterol improved.

After about four years of follow-ups, the effect on their weight remained and largely so did the effect on their blood sugar levels. Some still had normal blood sugar without medication. As such, they were cured, or at least symptom-free of their diabetes.

Nielsen's so-called Karlshamn Study was small and not randomized, but it was the first one.

Now there are nine randomized studies that compare low-carbohydrate with low-fat diets for people with type 2 diabetes. The results are clear.

5-0

A low-carbohydrate diet produced the best blood sugar in all nine studies. In five of them, the difference was clear (i.e., statistically significant).

But the win doesn't stop at the blood sugar level. It also produced better weight, blood pressure, and improved cholesterol levels in terms of generating more good cholesterol (HDL) and lower triglycerides. It is no accident that these five particular risk factors improved. They are intimately connected to type 2 diabetes and the Western disease.

The chart summarizes the winner in the study of weight, blood sugar (HbA1c), cholesterol (HDL, triglycerides), and blood pressure.

Study	Partici-pants	Months	Low-Carb	Low-Fat	Weight	HbA1c	HDL	TG	BT
Stern -04	54	12	6 %	55 %		LK*			
Daly -06	102	3	14 %	55 %	LK*	LK	LK*	LK	LK
Wolever -08	110	12	39 %	52 %	FS	LK	LK*	LK*	LK
Shai -08	31	24	4 % +	>50 %		LK			
Westman -08	84	6	4 %	55 %	LK*	LK*	LK*	LK	LK
Jönsson -09	13	3	32 %	42 %	LK*	LK*	LK*	LK*	LK*
Davis -09	105	12	4 % +	55 %	-	LK	LK*	LK	FS
Esposito -09	215	48	<50 %	>50 %	LK	LK*	LK*	LK*	LK
Elhayany -10	170	12	35 %	52 %	LK	LK*	LK*	LK*	

LK: E% carbohydrates for the low-carb group
FS: E% carbohydrates for the low-fat group
With a star: the difference between the groups was statistically significant
Greyish text: not statistically significant

Low-fat diets, today's dietary recommendations, perform the worst in all tests, even here. Not just for weight, but for blood pressure and other risk factors.

The media-friendly Professor Fredrik Nyström in Linköping is currently participating in a large Swedish study on diabetic diets. It is comparing low-carbohydrate diets to low-fat diets during a couple of years. We are expecting the results soon. I predict a huge breakthrough for the debate.

A convincing decade

One of the studies on diabetics was conducted by Dr. Eric Westman. I recently met him at a conference for American obesity doctors in Seattle. Dr. Westman is around fifty years old, but with a boyish appearance and a side part. He was once as scared of fat as other doctors. Until 1998, when he met several patients that had lost weight and improved their health metrics via the Atkins diet.

His curiosity piqued and he wrote to Dr. Atkins, who called him back. Dr. Westman asked: "Where's the science? I have read your book, but it only contains anecdotes." Atkins responded: "Come to my clinic. Why would I conduct a study when I already know the results?"

He flew to New York to meet with the controversial Dr. Atkins. Dr. Westman wanted to see if he was a lunatic, like his opponents claimed. Instead he was impressed. Dr. Atkins had met hordes of patients during his thirty years as a doctor and documented their positive results.

Dr. Westman decided that low-carbohydrate diets had earned the right to be studied more closely. He has now published a number of clinical studies with positive results. Many other researchers have done the same. In 1998 there barely existed any well-done scientific studies about low-carbohydrate diets. Now there are plenty. They show good results, and reality tells the same story.

When I was trapped in the United States after the conference (due to an Icelandic volcanic eruption), Dr. Westman invited me to visit him. I visited him for a couple of days in North Carolina and got to spend some time at his practice. He saw upward of thirty patients per day, often patients who were overweight with diabetes and elevated blood pressure. They were all advised to eat a low-carbohydrate diet. Patient after patient reported weight loss. During the visit, when someone had just lost 50 lbs (23 kg), Dr. Westman offered a complimentary piano concert and the song of his/her choice.[14]

What impressed me the most was not the weight. It was how patients were able to reduce their medication after almost each visit. First of all, they could reduce their blood sugar medication, often immediately at the time of the dietary change. Then they could continuously reduce their blood pressure medication and other things. They appeared to quickly become too healthy for their medicine.

I have seen similar results in my patients. I also receive daily emails from blog readers, often containing a thank-you for helping them lose weight and recover from diabetes. Real food can save many diabetics from terrible complications. It is frustrating to see how slowly the message about this new knowledge is spreading.

A federal fall forward

It is difficult for experts to do a complete turnaround. They need time. The change takes place in small steps. One clear example is when sbu, the Swedish council for medical evaluation, reviewed the diabetes dietary advice.

The Swedish usda used to be in charge of dietary advice for sick people. After a wise restructuring of the responsibility, that was transferred to the National Board of Health and Welfare. It has a better foundation in terms of medical competency. The National Board of Health and Welfare quickly realized that the issue of diabetic dietary recommendations was controversial and far from scientifically settled. Therefore, they transferred the issue to sbu.

---

14. The most surprising request they have received? "Fat Bottomed Girls" by Queen.

SBU collected a group of renowned experts to review the science. Their conclusion was published in the spring of 2010. They weren't able to conclude with certainty. There was "no scientific support" for today's low-fat dietary advice for diabetics. But they still didn't want to change them.

They noted the successful studies that had showed better results with low-carbohydrate diets. But the experts claimed that these studies were too small. During the ensuing debate, the experts wrote in *Dagens Media* magazine that changing dietary advice requires large and long studies.

In that context, that argument becomes exquisitely ironic. Why do we need perfect studies to change dietary advice when there are no such studies that prove established dietary recommendations?[15]

In SBU's defense, they have been humble. Professor Kjell Asplund, who led the evaluation, said: "We were surprised to find that the scientific basis for the long recommended diet is so weak." Professor Christian Berne, a leading expert on diabetes, said that the unsure situation produces a "significant freedom to give dietary advice that can be adjusted to each patient's wishes and expectations." They wrote that the lack of evidence for today's advice means we should be prepared to change the approach following future studies.

The system is somewhat sluggish. Change takes place painfully slowly. Fortunately you don't have to wait for those who are stuck in yesterday. You can eat exactly what you want. No one can stop you.

The freak of science

Despite resistance, Sweden is still the pioneer. The fact that diabetes diets are questioned and debated as openly as they are by doctors and

---

15. If you want to read about how SBU excluded so many studies that they could barely say anything about low-carbohydrate diets, see the reference section. It is predominantly interesting to study nerds.

in the media is unique. Sweden is years ahead of the rest of the world.

In the spring of 2010 I traveled to a rainy and cold Prague for a doctors' conference about controversial subjects within the diabetes community. At the stylish conference center at the Hilton, a thousand or so doctors gathered to learn more about reaching "consensus."

As usual, the pharmaceutical salesmen were posted outside the lecture rooms—beautiful women and well-dressed men. They were handing out pens, laser pointers, and pedometers with the name of new diabetes medications.

In the lecture rooms, only comfortable controversies were discussed. The fact that normalizing blood sugar with modern diabetes medication had shown to be fatal would have resulted in great confusion. But not enough confusion to question anything fundamental. Perhaps we are so far down the dead end that no one can see a way out.

The speakers seriously claimed that it could be dangerous for type 2 diabetics to have normal blood sugar. The fact that blood sugar can be reduced without medication or that the dietary recommendations are a part of the problem was not brought up. Professor after professor discussed whether or not they should change the color or size of the deck chairs. Meanwhile, Titanic kept sinking.

Why do knowledgeable, intelligent people fail to see a solution? It is not as unfathomable as it looks. They are trapped in a contrived model that was necessary for keeping the theory about the dangers of fat. This is what it looks like, somewhat simplified: If you eat too much and run too little, you become fat. Body fat leaks into the blood and produces, in a complicated way, reduced sensitivity to insulin. If the body cannot produce enough insulin, the blood sugar rises and you get type 2 diabetes.

That way, the cause for elevated blood sugar can be blamed on fatty food (which doesn't raise the blood sugar) while carbohydrates, which do raise the blood sugar, go free. Clever, huh? But the theory is a scientific freak.[16]

If the resistance to insulin had been the main problem and if it had been caused by being overweight, the solution would be to lose weight, which is difficult when the elevated blood sugar blocks the fat burning. To reduce the insulin, diabetics need to lose weight, which the high insulin blocks. That is the hopeless catch-22. No wonder diabetics keep getting sicker and heavier.

The solution is liberating. With fewer carbohydrates, the blood sugar and insulin levels decrease. Low insulin increases your fat-burning process and you lose weight. The insulin resistance decreases, resulting in further weight loss. You end up in a positive cycle. You become healthier and thinner without hunger.

The old theory is said to be the reason why today's diabetes treatment kills type 2 diabetics. They usually have an abnormally high level of insulin in their blood. The old theory blames it on sensitivity to insulin. The treatment is more insulin.

How can you treat someone with elevated insulin with more insulin? That is like treating hyperthyroidism, too much of the thyroid hormone, with more thyroid hormone. Or a cortisol-producing tumor with cortisone pills. A doctor that behaved that way would be stripped of his or her license.

Seriously, when you use insulin to treat type 2 diabetics who already had high insulin to begin with, are you surprised that they die more quickly?

---

16. That can quickly be counter-argued. The theory assumes that obesity (via insulin resistance) is the culprit that produced high blood sugar. But when a diabetic starts a low-carbohydrate diet, his or her blood sugar often normalizes within days, long before your weight has changed. That has even been proved in studies. The same thing can be seen in diabetics who undergo a gastric bypass surgery where the blood sugar is quickly normalized, before the weight is adjusted. After the stomach has been disabled, you cannot eat a large amount of carbohydrates.

The obesity cannot be the reason for high blood sugar in type 2 diabetics. The blood sugar can be normalized without the body weight having had time to adjust.

Stable blood sugar

We should also mention type 1 diabetics. They have a different problem—they lack their own insulin. It can be replaced with insulin injections. That's why they are said to be able to eat anything.

It's not quite that simple. Healthy bodies have a meticulously regulated insulin production to control the blood sugar. Type 1 diabetics have three tricky tasks. They have to predict the volume of necessary insulin and how well the food and injected insulin will be absorbed.

They can become quite skilled at it, but without a sixth sense, predictions are never perfect. The more carbohydrates type 1 diabetics eat, the more their blood sugar rises, and the more insulin is required. That provides a fluctuating blood sugar with risk of severe dips.

What would happen on a low-carbohydrate diet? Jörgen Vesti Nielsen, chief of medicine in Karlshamn, Sweden, wanted an answer to that question as well. He let twenty-four type 1 diabetics try a moderately strict low-carbohydrate diet (16 percent carbohydrates).

The test resulted in stabilized blood sugar. The number of blood sugar dips fell by more than 80 percent The average blood sugar (HbA1c) improved significantly from 7.5 to 6.4, and they could almost cut their meal insulin in half. Even their cholesterol levels improved.

Here is a blood sugar curve that shows the dietary change of one of the patients over the course of three weeks:

Blood sugar

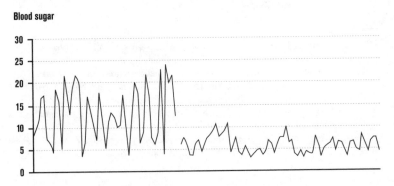

Blood sugar

On the left: twelve days with regular food. On the right: ten days on a low-carbohydrate diet and adjusted (lowered) insulin doses. Which blood sugar curve do you prefer?

Type 1 diabetics who have achieved a somewhat stable blood sugar with a lot of carbohydrates are experts at insulin dosage. With a low-carbohydrate diet, they would probably achieve a record-breaking curve.

I have met many type 1 diabetics who have tried it. They usually say the same thing—they achieve a more stable blood sugar and have an easier time predicting insulin doses. Sometimes they can manage without a dose with their meal when they consume few carbohydrates, without the blood sugar rising significantly. A common side effect of reduced insulin doses is a reduction of potential extra weight.[17]

"Why obsess about the sugar?"

I was recently at a two-day conference on obesity. During the breaks, they served coffee in the exhibition hall, where companies were present to sell their products. I obtained a fancy brochure from one of the pharmaceutical companies that sell diabetes medicine. The brochure was called "Food and Diabetes."

The cover featured a beautiful young woman holding a big

---

17. How does it work in the long run? The American doctor and type 1 diabetic Richard K. Bernstein knows. For decades, he has advocated for a low-carbohydrate diet. He has tried and seen the effects firsthand, and he has seen thousands of patients through his practice in Manhattan. He trained to become a doctor late in life to spread the knowledge. At seventy-six, Bernstein is still working. His book *The Diabetes Solution* is the most comprehensive book about low-carbohydrate diets and diabetes.

fruit basket with a big thumbs-up. Fruit is sweet. Fruit contains approximately 10 percent sugar, just as much as a can of Coke. Is sugar good for diabetics? I doubt it. But the inside of the brochure was worse.

Good food for diabetes, it claims, is food that slowly raises the blood sugar. Turns out, that is the type of food that in 1917 was absolutely forbidden for diabetics, such as pasta, rice, potatoes, and bread. But sugar also works, according to the new brochure. It talks about how flour raises the blood sugar as much as sugar does. The quote said, "We allow flour. Why should we then obsess about sugar?"

Their life-threatening dietary advice makes diabetics sicker. Good food for diabetics is not food that raises the blood sugar slowly and significantly. It is actually food that *doesn't* raise the blood sugar: meat, fish, eggs, and butter. The fact that flour is just as bad as sugar doesn't mean it can be consumed in unlimited quantities; both should actually be avoided.

Patients receive sickening dietary advice from personnel that probably don't know better. But I cannot help but wonder about the brochures. The pharmaceutical companies have to know that the more carbohydrates a diabetic eats, the more insulin and other medications are required. They sell the drugs and hand out fancy brochures with extremely carbohydrate-happy dietary advice. Diabetics who follow the recommendations will need more medicine and the companies will make even more money. Does that sound like a conspiracy theory? Or is it too naïve to think otherwise?

If you could compensate for blood sugar-raising dietary advice with expensive drugs, the brochures would simply affect taxpayers and insurance costs. When the medications are potentially fatal, the problem is larger.

The madness's delicate end

But blood sugar-raising carbohydrates and more blood sugar-reducing medications is not the solution to type 2 diabetes. Science is.

Unfortunately, the healthcare industry is maltreating Sweden's 350,000 diabetics. This maltreatment unnecessarily makes patients sicker instead of healthier. There is no nicer way of putting it.

Some defend the obsolete dietary advice, saying, "Diabetics have the right to eat just like everybody else." Those who say that perhaps think they are doing something good, but they aren't. It is a pat on the head.

If some people *want* to try a low-carbohydrate diet, if some diabetics would rather refrain from the pastry with their coffee than risk blindness or amputation, it is up to him or her. Healthcare professionals shouldn't make that decision for anyone. What diabetics are indeed entitled to is accurate information and the opportunity to make their own choices.

Once we abandon the failed fear of fat, we can see clearly again. Evolution, countless stories from those who have tried the diet, and a growing number of scientific studies, give us the answer. The answer for diabetics is a low-carbohydrate diet. It produces normal blood sugar, a reduced need for medication, and better health.

You don't need to return to lard and cucumbers like diabetics hundreds of years ago did. Not at all. The future of diabetic diets can be served in luxurious restaurants as well as easily and significantly cheaper in your home.

You can eat meat and vegetables cooked in butter, with a scrumptious cream sauce, and a glass of wine. You can enjoy eating until you are full while becoming healthier and leaner. I wish you all the best.

Note the absence of purified sugar or starch

Now the time has come to seal the deal. Your weight and blood sugar is only the beginning. This is bigger. Sometimes you have to abandon preconceived notions to see the road ahead. Like Vilhjalmur Stefansson. He left civilization and returned a hundred years later as a changed man. His story follows here.

CHAPTER SEVEN

The Western diseases

R esearch has shown clear connections. Obese people and everyone with type 2 diabetes have an increased risk of cancer, dementia, gallstone, gout, cavities, heart disease, and so on.

What does that mean? We are closing in on the answer, via a story from one of civilization's coldest and most remote locations.

Healthier than ever

Vilhjalmur Stefansson didn't like fish. He had avoided fish his whole life. Now he had nothing else to eat for a whole winter.

It was 1906, and he had tagged along on his first expedition to northern Canada. He was twenty-seven years old, university educated, and excited for an adventure. His goal was to study the primitive Eskimos, the Inuit, who lived there. He succeeded and was pretty much adopted by one of the families during that year. He lived in a house constructed from wood and clay with one room—along with twenty-two other people.

Breakfast at 7:00 a.m. consisted of freshly defrosted winter fish (raw), lunch at 11:00 a.m. was the same thing, and dinner at 4:00 p.m. was boiled fish. As a night meal, they ate leftovers from dinner: fish.

During the days, the men and half of the women were out fishing in the cold. When they returned at dinner time, the home was heated enough to feel like a sauna.

A couple of months later, Stefansson hadn't just gotten used to the food, he actually liked it. Throughout the winter, he ate almost nothing but fish and water. Afterwards, he felt physically and mentally healthier than ever.

Stefansson returned numerous times to the Arctic plains throughout the next couple of decades. Each time he subsisted on the food that was available: fish and meat (from seal or polar bear). No vegetables or grains could be cultivated in the cold. In sum, he lived off of almost nothing but meat for more than five years during increasingly longer expedition cycles.

Eventually he received some recognition for the books he wrote about his adventurous trips. He was also very controversial for advocating a low-carbohydrate diet based on animal meat. He recognized how good it made him feel and how the excess fat quickly disappeared from his body.

Despite years among the Inuit, Stefansson never saw a fat person while they still subsisted on their traditional food in the beginning of the twentieth century. Not a single person—they were all thin. The transformation came when they started adding Western food to their diet.

Indian blood

Let's leap forward a hundred years to the present day. The remainders of Canada's indigenous population, including the Inuit, have had to abandon their traditional lifestyles. They don't subsist purely on meat and fish anymore. They live off of cheap Western food, filled with sugar and starch.

Stefansson, who died in 1962, wouldn't have recognized it. Gone are the people who never experienced obesity, whose language didn't even have a word for "diabetes." On the contrary, obesity and diabetes are now endemic to the population; they have become common.

All of the diseases that normally arrive at the same time are now common: heart disease, cancer, dementia, gout, and gallstones.

The Canadian doctor Jay Wortman wants to change things, and he believes that he knows how to do it. By changing a society in front of TV cameras.

Dr. Wortman is half Native American. You can tell from his facial features and the color of his skin. His eyes look somewhat saddened and the grayish hair conjures an image of a wise man.

A couple of years ago, like many others, he came to an unsolicited insight. As a doctor, he had believed he was immune to the diseases he diagnosed and treated in others, despite the fact that many in his own family had suffered from type 2 diabetes. He long dismissed the fatigue, excess weight, the required midnight visits to the bathroom, increased thirst, the need to squint to read the TV news, and the blood pressure that had risen to levels that required medical attention. After all, he was approaching fifty. Wasn't that inevitable at his age?

Suddenly Dr. Wortman realized what was wrong. He had the classic symptoms of diabetes. It was during a weekend, and he was at home. He brought a blood sugar-measuring device into the bathroom. He only had to prick his finger and analyze the small drop of blood to know the answer. His blood sugar had skyrocketed.

Shocked, he didn't know what to do. To allow himself to investigate further, he decided to buy himself some time. He decided to not eat anything that would worsen his condition. He stopped eating carbohydrates. He barely knew anything about low-carbohydrate diets; it was thought of as a temporary solution, until he could start his real treatment.

But something unexpected occurred. His blood sugar stabilized almost immediately. He started losing close to a pound per day. The rest of his symptoms quickly decreased. He started seeing clearly again, the nightly bathroom visits and thirst disappeared, he regained energy, and he felt a lot better.

His wife explained to him that he was on an Atkins diet, something he hadn't realized. She had previously bought the Atkins book to lose post-pregnancy weight. Jay Wortman had dismissed it as a fad diet that would hardly work in the long run. Now he started studying.

His work as a doctor focused on the health of the Canadian indigenous population. He was highly aware of the fact that while the diabetes epidemic had spread across Canada, the situation among the indigenous was disastrous. The precursor to diabetes, obesity, and metabolic syndrome (more about that soon) was extremely common. These epidemics had a catastrophic impact on the indigenous communities, and their healthcare cost more than they could afford.

While a dietary change solved his own health issues, he started to look at the indigenous people's health crisis from a new perspective. In his work he often traveled to indigenous communities. He started to ask them, especially the elders, about their traditional food. It turned out to contain very few carbohydrates: fish, seafood, moose, deer, and more, in addition to berries and seasonal plants.

It was different now: bread, potatoes, and pasta salad were common dinner sides; pastries for dessert, and accompanied by soda or juice. Dr. Wortman couldn't help but wonder: would they see the same effect as he did if they returned to their traditional food? Would they become healthy?

He contacted doctors in the United States who had long researched and used a low-carbohydrate diet with positive results, such as Dr. Eric Westman, Dr. Steve Phinney, and Dr. Mary Vernon. With their help, he planned a study.

The documented return of health

A couple of years later, Canadian TV aired a documentary about his study, which became the most talked-about film of the year. The title was MY BIG FAT DIET—SMALL TOWN WINS THE WEIGHT RACE. The population of Albert Bay, an isolated former fishing village, is comprised mostly of descendants of the indigenous population. The prevalence of obesity, diabetes, and metabolic syndrome is about four times higher than the already-high Canadian average.

Jay Wortman and his associates got almost a hundred residents to try to refrain from sugar and starch for one year and instead eat more meat, fish, vegetables, and other low-carbohydrate foods. What convinced many of them was the fact that they were returning to the same diet their ancestors had eaten.

The only grocery store in the village noticed the transformation. Egg sales tripled, but what increased the most was a specific vegetable. As cauliflower replaced more carbohydrate-rich foods (like rice and pasta), the sales increased about five times.

The participants were tracked for a year by a doctor and a nurse. The health results all pointed in the same direction, regardless of where you looked. People's weights dropped an average of 22 lbs (10 kg), the blood sugar and cholesterol levels improved significantly, and many could reduce their blood pressure and diabetes medications. Without the modern food, the new diseases started to retract. Health returned.

But Dr. Wortman hasn't just helped others regain health. I met him eight years after his dietary change, and he was still thin and healthy. His blood sugar and other blood tests are still normal without medication.

Wortman has two small children today. He should be able to see them graduate without diabetes having stolen his vision, feet, or life. He has a good likelihood of seeing his children grow up and have grandkids, and will be able to approach retirement with dignity. Jay Wortman has escaped the Western disease.

A sick world

Canada is a good example. In a couple of centuries, the Western disease spread across the world, like we saw in chapter one. More countries started to eat like us, get sick like us, and die like us. The same diseases spread everywhere the new food appeared.

Before our modern medical knowledge started to accelerate, the diseases were prevalent across the globe, in all countries. These diseases, which had previously been rare or unknown, became normalized. Diabetes, obesity, gout, gallstones, cancer, and so on—the Western diseases.

Coca-Cola and white flour are omnipresent today. We cannot turn back time. We can no longer study the health of people who lived before they were developed. But we can read the accounts from people who were there. Those who realized, those who reacted. They were often Western doctors who worked in colonized countries. What they saw the local populations go through in a matter of a couple of decades was horrifying. They were suddenly afflicted with our diseases.

But today we have access to something else. Today, modern science can start to explain why it happened. We now have knowledge about the body's function down to the molecular level, which provides us with fascinating insight into what went wrong.

Heart attacks, difficulties in conceiving children, acne, enlarged prostates, and dementia. Diseases that are regarded as part of life in the Western world. They are all strongly tied to obesity and diabetes. They seem to be related. More and more things are showing that they are different manifestations of the same bodily malfunction.

Let's start with the big killer, the one Ancel Keys erroneously thought was caused by fat in the 1950s—heart disease. Heart attacks. Today we know that there was never a correlation between fat or saturated fat and heart disease. So what is the cause?

In retrospect, the picture is clearer. Ancel Keys found that in some select rich countries, people consumed more fat and had more heart disease than in poorer undeveloped countries. That turned out to be a red herring. But there was something that had the same, if not a stronger correlation. In the rich countries, people also consumed more sugar and white flour.

Now it is time to see how it is all really connected. What Keys never realized.

The big killer

In the West, cardiovascular diseases such as heart attacks and strokes have long been the most fatal diseases. Four out of ten

Swedes still die from heart diseases. With a significantly reduced number of smokers, more preventative medications, and better healthcare, many live a long life before dying. But perhaps you want to avoid the disease entirely and not require the medications.

What is the cause of heart disease? There have been plenty of theories. Like the 1950s theory about dangerously elevated cholesterol. But most people who suffer heart attacks don't have high cholesterol. It wasn't that simple. The next chapter straightens out the more complicated relationship between cholesterol and heart disease. That's the last piece of the puzzle, but there are some remaining ones before that.

Cardiovascular disease means that the walls of the arteries get clogged by plaque. This can make the artery too tight for blood to pass, which results in a painful lack of oxygen in the tissues downstream. Clogged arteries that lead to the heart cause angina, chest pain, as the heart struggles to get more blood and oxygen.

The worst thing is that plaque can rupture and create a wound in the artery wall. That causes the blood to coagulate around the wound and create a scab in the wall. That can clog the artery and block the blood flow. The tissue downstream receives no oxygen and dies. If the artery in question goes to the heart, you suffer a heart attack. If it is located in the brain, you suffer a stroke. The bigger the artery, the worse the result.

What causes the disease in the arteries? Nowadays, they agree that a couple of different factors collaborate to increase the risk. Most of them seem to have something in common.

In the largest observational study about this, INTERHEART, they examined almost thirty thousand people around the world. Half of them had just had their first heart attack, the other half were people without the disease. Then they compared the two groups. What signifies the ones who have developed heart disease? What is more common among them than in healthy people?

Six things are different. These things are more common among people with heart disease:

1. Abdominal obesity
2. Diabetes
3. High blood pressure
4. An abnormal lipid distribution (high apo ratio[18])
5. Smoking
6. Stress

Smokers and people with stressful lives more often suffer from heart attacks. That is good to know, but falls outside the main theme of this book. However, the first four things, those that are affected by what you eat, they *are* the topic of this book. They are symptoms of the Western disease.

The core of the disease: metabolic syndrome

Memorize the expression "metabolic syndrome." You will hear about it a lot. That is the medical term for the Western disease.

Since the middle of the twentieth century, a funny phenomenon has become increasingly apparent. Some diseases and risk factors for heart disease are not randomly distributed among the populations. Not at all. They seem to connect with each other.

If you suffer from abdominal obesity, you are more likely to get diabetes. People with high blood pressure often have abnormal lipid profiles. If you have type 2 diabetes, you almost always have a big belly and high blood pressure. Why? Perhaps because obesity, diabetes, and heart disease all share the same root cause.

The risk factors are connected; they can be found in the same types of people. That's true for many other diseases, not just heart disease. It is reminiscent of a Bible quote, Matthew 13:12, "For to the one who has, more will be given, and he will have an abundance, but from the one who has not, even what he has will be taken away."

---

18. The apo ratio is a newer and more accurate cholesterol measurement. Read more about it in the next chapter.

Those who are already sick get more diseases and die prematurely. Healthy people continue to stay healthy. They often seem thin and happy as well. The world is unfair when it comes to health. Now the causes are starting to become clearer.

Metabolic syndrome formally means that someone has three of these five risk factors simultaneously:

1. *Abdominal obesity:* Waist circumference > 40 in (102 cm) men, > 35 in (88 cm) women
2. *High blood sugar:* Fasting blood sugar > 110 MG/DL
3. *High blood pressure:* Below 130/85, or on blood pressure medication
4. *Abnormal lipid profile 1:* Triglycerides > 150 MG/DL
5. *Abnormal lipid profile 2:* HDL cholesterol < 45 MG/DL men, < 1.3 women

Metabolic syndrome has become horrifyingly common. In the United States, more than every third adult already has it, and more than every other elderly person. Even more people show some sign of it. In Sweden, the majority of elderly people already takes blood pressure medication and every third elderly person takes medicine for cholesterol.

Metabolic syndrome, the Western disease, is now extremely common. How dangerous is it?

118 cigarettes a day

People with metabolic syndrome have an increased risk for almost all types of endemic disease—heart disease, cancer, dementia, and all other types of unpleasantries.

It is difficult to know exactly how dangerous metabolic syndrome actually is. You can get a rough estimate by playing with statistics from the INTERHEART study.

To make it more concrete, I am comparing it to smoking. Smokers more frequently suffer from heart attacks, and the risk increases with the number of cigarettes per day. If you smoke ten cigarettes a day, the risk doubles. With a pack, twenty cigarettes, the risk quadruples, and with two packs, the risk increases eight times.

How much do you have to smoke for it to be as dangerous as metabolic syndrome? Here is an estimate based on observational data:

RISK FACTOR	THE INCREASED RISK EQUALS
Abdominal obesity	7 cigarettes a day
Diabetes	12 cigarettes a day
High blood pressure	9 cigarettes a day
Abnormal lipid profile	16 cigarettes a day

That is the risk increase with a risk factor. That would be bad enough. But the risk increases aren't just added together if you have more than one. They exacerbate the effects of each other. The more risk factors you have, the higher the risk is for heart disease. What happens if you have all of them?

RISK FACTOR	THE RISK INCREASE EQUALS
All four at the same time	118 cigarettes a day

In sum, a complete metabolic syndrome may be as dangerous as smoking six packs a day. Like chain-smoking three cigarettes at a time.

If you are afflicted with this, the question is evident: can anything be done about it? Something that can immediately improve all of these risk factors? A way of killing two birds with one stone? The answer is yes.

Here is the perfect correlation that can still leave me breathless.

The risk factors that are associated with metabolic syndrome are practically identical to the diet-related risk factors for heart disease. But that's not all.

The exact same risk factors are the same that time after time are proven to be ameliorated with a low-carbohydrate diet.

A perfect correlation

A low-carbohydrate diet reduces your abdominal obesity, lowers your blood sugar and blood pressure, and improves your lipid profile (measured as HDL, triglycerides, or with an apo ratio). It improves the entire metabolic syndrome.

The chart summarizes the winner in studies on weight, blood sugar (HbA1c), cholesterol (HDL, triglycerides) and blood pressure.

Study	Partici-pants	Months	Low Carb group	Low Fat group	Weight	HbA1c	HDL	Tri-glycer-ides	Blood pressure
Brehm -03	53	6	4–12 %	55 %	LK*		LK	LK*	LK
Foster -03	63	12	4 % +	60 %	LK		LK*	LK*	LK
Samaha -03	132	6	6 %	55 %	LK*	LK		LK*	
Sondike -03	30	3	4–8 %	55 %	LK*		LK	LK	
Aude -04	60	3	10–28 %	55 %	LK*		LK	LK	
Volek -04	31	1,5	<10 %	60 %	LK*				
Meckling -04	31	2,5	12 %	55 %	LK		LK*	LK	LK
Yancy -04	120	6	4 % +	55 %	LK*		LK*	LK*	LK
Stern -04	132	12	6 %	55 %	LK	LK*	LK*	LK*	
Nickols-R -05	28	1,5	4 % +	60 %	LK*				
Dansinger -05	80	12	4–10 %	55 %	FS		LK	FS	FS
Truby -06	212	6	4 % +	55 %	LK				LK
Gardner-07	153	12	4–10 %	55–60 %	LK*		LK*	LK*	LK*
Ebbeling -07	73	18	40 %	55 %	LK		LK*	LK	LK
Shai 08	213	24	4 % +	>50 %	LK*	LK	LK*	LK*	
Sacks -09	811	24	35, 45 %	55–65 %	LK		LK	LK	FS
Brinkworth -09	118	12	4 %	46 %	LK		LK*	LK*	
Frisch -09	200	12	<40 %	>55 %	LK		LK	LK	LK*
Yancy -10	146	11	4 % +	55 % + Xenical	LK	LK	LK	LK	LK*
Foster -10	307	24	4 % +	55 %	FS		LK*	FS	LK*
Krebs -10	46	3	4 %	55 %	LK*		LK	LK	
Meta analyses									
Nordmann -06	5 studies	6			LK*		LK*	LK*	LK
Hession -09	13 studies	12			LK*		LK*	LK*	LK*

Low Carb group: the column indicates the amount of energy percent of carbohydrates in the diet of the low carbohydrate group

Low fat group: the column indicates the amount of energy percent of carbohydrates in the diet of the low fat group

A star: the difference between the groups were statistically significant

Plus sign: the amount of carbohydrates increases somewhat with time

Grayish text: not a statistically significant result

The exact improvements have been illustrated in well-conducted randomized studies (see the chart on the previous page).

It is time to follow the logical path behind that thought.

If a low-carbohydrate diet improves the risk factors, are sugar and starch, the new foods, the cause of heart disease?

That is a revolutionary possibility. But heart disease and its risk factors, such as obesity and diabetes, are just the beginning. When the sugar and starch spread across the world about a hundred years ago, suddenly an array of new diseases became commonplace. Today's endemic diseases.

These diseases are connected to the metabolic syndrome. If you suffer from metabolic syndrome, you have an increased risk of getting them. Is it then possible that they all have a common root cause?

Healthier arteries

First, more about heart disease. Science has actually come farther than just studying risk factors.

Major, high-quality studies have tested low-fat diets with disastrous results. Time after time, it has failed to prevent heart disease. In the biggest study, WHI, people with a heart condition actually became sick from low-fat diets. The faith in low-fat products was obviously a mistake.

The challenger, the low-carbohydrate diet, results in improved risk factors. However, the effect on the arteries has not been thoroughly examined yet. We don't know the full positive effect yet. But a couple of new studies have provided interesting results.

In 2004, Harvard published a fascinating and well-conducted study. It was received with absolute silence. No one knew how to handle the results. If fat were dangerous, the result of the study was inexplicable, so it was ignored.

The study tracked a couple of hundred women with heart disease. Their coronary arteries were x-rayed, and they repeated the examination three years later. They could see whether or not the arteries had become more clogged.

What shocked many was the connection to what the women had been eating. The *less* saturated fat they had eaten, the *more* their arteries had clogged. They became sicker when they ate what was recommended. The correlation was self-evident, too strong to be dismissed. It was impossible to reconcile with the belief that saturated fat is life-threatening. Therefore, the study could only be ignored.

Now that saturated fat was found not guilty, we can see clearly. The problem is that if you are unnecessarily scared of natural fat, you eat more of something else, something more dangerous, something that can really cause heart disease. The correlation with carbohydrates was just as strong, but was going the opposite way.

The fewer the carbohydrates the women had consumed, the healthier their arteries became.

Similar findings were soon repeated. The largest observational study that examined this is the Nurse's Health study. It has tracked eighty thousand American nurses for a couple of decades. The correlation between carbohydrate intake and heart diseases among them was interesting enough to be published in one of the most renowned journals of them all, the *New England Journal of Medicine*. The nurses that voluntarily chose to eat fewer simple carbohydrates, like sugar and starch, had significantly reduced their risk of heart disease.

The results in these studies were clear. But they are observational studies. They aren't the most accurate studies science can offer, the fairest comparison. The best is a randomized intervention study that examines the effects on the arteries. Now such a study exists.

The large Israeli study led by Iris Shai in 2008 demonstrated more weight loss and better cholesterol levels after two years on a low-carbohydrate diet, compared to a low-fat diet. That was never mentioned in the weight chapter. But that's not all. In 2010, they published the results of the participants' neck arteries, measured with an ultrasound.

Those who had followed a low-carbohydrate diet not only improved their weight and cholesterol. Something also happened with the clogging of their arteries. It decreased. The arteries looked visibly better after two years on a low-carbohydrate diet.

A low-carbohydrate diet improves all the risk factors of metabolic syndrome. It results in healthier arteries and fewer instances of heart disease.

Let's now turn to the other new Western diseases. Our modern endemic diseases. There are many to choose from, like cancer and dementia. But let's start with another one. One that might be completely unexpected.

An anti-seizure effect

Charlie Abrahams had his first epileptic seizure when he was one year old. Epilepsy is characterized by episodes of abnormal brain activity. Often, like in Charlie's case, the cause is unknown. Soon, his parents found themselves in the middle of a nightmare. Little Charlie increasingly suffered seizures with muscle cramps and unconsciousness, upwards of a hundred times a day.

Charlie's parents sought out the best doctors they could find. They tried all available medications, but they weren't effective enough. Not even drugging him to a zombie-esque state eliminated the seizures. The constant episodes risked making Charlie permanently brain-damaged or mentally handicapped.

It was a race against time. His parents let him undergo brain surgery, wherein they removed a part of the brain from where the seizures appeared to derive. But the attacks kept occurring. The doctors had no solution. The parents were desperate. Charlie's dad read every possible book about epilepsy. And one day, in a medical library, he found something. Something no one had told him.

It was a book about epilepsy that mentioned a diet that claimed to cure half of the children that had tried it, a diet that had been successfully used since 1921. The doctors that used it worked at Johns Hopkins Hospital in Baltimore, one of America's most prestigious hospitals. Charlie's dad was astounded. Was it possible? How had no one told them about this possibility? His doctor recommended against it, but he took Charlie to the other side of the United States, to the Children's Hospital in Baltimore, and met the author of the book, Dr. John Friedman.

Charlie Abrahams got to try it. They removed all of his medication and fed him the specific diet that mostly consisted of fat. The frequency of his seizures dropped dramatically. After a couple of days, they had been entirely eliminated. Charlie had returned and didn't even need medication. It was like night and day. But the story doesn't end there.

His parents reacted as expected. They were happy about the result, but angry at the same time.[19] Why hadn't they found out about this before? Charlie was just one of many similar cases in Baltimore. How could numerous epilepsy-stricken children be cured there, while others didn't even hear about it?

One reason is that there isn't as much money in the diet treatment business as in the pharmaceutical industry. The dietary alternative is actually discouraged. Despite spectacular results, it was seen as dangerous alternative medicine. It was difficult to spread that knowledge. But Charlie's parents weren't just anybody.

---

19. That reaction is common for people who successfully try a low-carbohydrate diet. Often they have a difficult time succeeding with a low-fat diet for excess weight or diabetes. Then they do the complete opposite and become healthier and thinner. Of course, the happiness is the main feeling. But it is often mixed with anger toward those who have given them bad advice (albeit well-meaning) or against the entire system. Especially when they realize there are no valid reasons for fearing fat.

They had resources and contacts. They could change things. They started in 1994.

Epilepsy

Almost every hundredth Swede suffers from epilepsy today, and the reason is often unknown. It could be one of the Western diseases. Standard treatment is medication that reduces the risk of having a seizure. The medications all have side effects. They impair nerve signals, which makes the brain function sub-optimally. Yet they are preferred over constant seizures. But what if there is another alternative?

As you now know, it exists. That alternative has quickly become more accepted—eating very few carbohydrates and more fat. That eliminates blood sugar peaks. It makes the blood sugar more stable and instead fuels the brain with fat.[20] In some way, it also calms the brain so that epileptic attacks are reduced in frequency and severity.

A strict low-carbohydrate diet is no longer controversial in the treatment of children with severe epilepsy. A couple of new and high-quality studies show great effects. They traditionally use a special diet with an extremely high ratio of fat. In recent years they have tried more natural and tastier food. A version of the Atkins diet based on natural food, meat and fish, vegetables, and natural fats like butter has also shown demonstrated effects on sick children.

Why has the low-carbohydrate diet had such a quick breakthrough? How did it grow from a suspicious alternative medicine to an accepted standard treatment in only a decade? One reason is Charlie's dad, Jim.

Abrahams was a successful film director in Hollywood. He was predominantly known for the eighties and nineties comedies *Air-*

---

20. Technically the brain then partially utilizes ketone bodies, an energy molecule in the blood that is formed from fat in the liver. It is called ketosis and is normal if you haven't consumed carbohydrates in a while and thus experience increased fat metabolism.

Unfortunately, there are plenty of misconceptions around the harmless ketosis. See the chapter "Questions & Answers" later in the book.

plane!, *The Naked Gun*, and *Hot Shots*. But now he can feel proud over the amount of smiles he has generated.

He started the organization *The Charlie Foundation*, which has effectively spread the message about the effects of low-carbohydrate diets on child epilepsy. Parents everywhere started requesting the treatment, which therefore spread to more hospitals.

Jim Abrahams directed a movie based on a similar true story, called *First Do No Harm*, starring Meryl Streep.[21] You watch her deliver a passionate speech on the organization's website. You can also watch TV shows in the US and interviews with doctors talking about the astonishingly positive results, and read numerous moving stories from parents and children. I highly recommend a visit to the website, even if you don't suffer from epilepsy. See www.charliefoundation.org.

One question remains. Why just children? Recently the same diet was tested on thirty adults with epilepsy. They more or less had daily epileptic seizures, some almost every hour. They had each tried dozens of different medications, and some had even undergone brain surgery without eliminating their seizures.

Despite this, about half of the participants significantly improved when they followed the Atkins diet. The number of seizures halved, and some of the participants even lost up to 15 lbs (7 kg). Some eliminated their seizures entirely. Those are some impressive results from a dietary change, especially considering how sick and difficult to treat they were before.

---

21. The child on whom the movie is based, Tim, had severe epilepsy with around 150 to 200 seizures per day. Despite countless doctors and medications, no one could help him. In the end he was committed to an intensive care facility for months with constant attacks despite eight different medicines and a Valium IV (perhaps he simultaneously had a fructose IV in the other arm).

The mother heard of the treatment in Baltimore. She had to "steal" her son from the hospital and transport him directly there with the help of a nurse and a retired doctor. The results of the low-carbohydrate diet were everything they had dreamed about. That took place several decades ago. Tim has yet to experience another epileptic seizure.

The study was small, but still the largest dietary treatment of adult epileptics to date. Conversely, there are plenty of studies about medications. Unfortunately, the drug business has all the money.

The last question is of course this: why is it helping only the most severely sick? People with less severe epilepsy should be able to become even healthier. Perhaps they don't have to be as thorough about their food. They should also be informed of the fact that they might be able to become seizure-free by avoiding sugar and starch.

Medication for epilepsy may result in dizziness, deteriorated memory, and difficulty thinking straight. Many of them even cause weight gain. If I suffered from epilepsy, I would want to know that a low-carbohydrate diet might be an option.

Of course, there is no guarantee that it helps everybody. But eating real food without sugar or starch is harmless, contrary to medicines and brain surgery. Why not try it today? When we leave the unnecessary fear of fat behind, we are all good to go. And epilepsy is just the beginning.

Calm stomachs

One of the most common diseases in the world is called Irritable Bowel Syndrome (IBS). That translates into a sensitive digestive system. More than every tenth Swede suffers from it today, and it can generate abdominal pain, gas, bloating, and interchanging loose and hard feces.

No one claims to know the cause of this very common disease. There is no effective medicine for it. Yet we know what causes gas problems. Pea soup and brown beans, for example. Why? Fiber and other carbohydrates in the food that isn't absorbed in the small intestine continue to the colon. There, they become food for bacteria, which ferments it and produces gas. Excess gas results in stomachaches, bloating, and flatulence.

You may wonder what happens when you follow a low-carbohydrate diet, even if you are careful with fiber-rich vegetables. According to experiences from patients, friends, and blog readers, the answer is evident—a calmer digestive system with less gas (or none). Almost all seem to experience the same thing. Yet only one scientific study has examined a low-carbohydrate diet in relation to a sensitive digestive system.

Seventeen people with sensitive intestines and severe diarrhea discomfort recently tested a strict low-carbohydrate diet (maximum twenty grams per day) for four weeks. Out of the thirteen that completed the whole study, all got better. They had more normal feces, fewer stomachaches and better quality of life. Perhaps something you want to experience?

A less common digestive condition is gluten intolerance. A protein in the grains activates the body's immune system, which harms the intestine. It can result in diarrhea, fatigue, and nutrition deficiencies. A strict low-carbohydrate diet cuts out grains, which makes a gluten-intolerant person symptom-free. It is not even controversial.

It's not just discomfort in the lower regions of the stomach, the intestine, that is common today. A lot of people also have issues with the stomach itself, often called gastritis. Or they suffer from heartburn—stomach acid that leaks into the esophagus. Most people have experienced it.

Pills for heartburn that reduce the stomach acid are one of the most lucrative medications ever. The medication Prilosec (omeprazole) earned enormous amounts of money and made the Swedish company Astra (now called AstraZeneca) one of the world's largest pharmaceutical companies. During the 1990s, Prilosec was one of the world's most sold pharmaceuticals, before the patent ran out. Now a generic version can be purchased more cheaply and over the counter in pharmacies.

You may wonder if heartburn is also one of the Western diseases? Maybe, maybe not. But obesity increases the pressure on the stomach and can make the issues worse. Weight loss helps.

Oftentimes, something else seems to happen faster than that, before the weight has changed. I won't go into uncertain experiences from people who have tried a low-carbohydrate diet. The effect on heartburn is not as clear as on digestive issues. I just want to mention a small study which is, to the best of my knowledge, the only one that has examined this issue.

Eight obese patients with severe heartburn tested a strict low-carbohydrate diet (maximum twenty grams per day). Their esophagus pH level was measured prior to the study, and then again six days into it. Both their symptoms and pH levels improved significantly during that short period of time. Without sweet food, they were no longer as acidic.

Calmer stomachs are great, but women have more to gain.

Bearded ladies

No one wants to be overweight with acne and a patchy beard. Especially not women. Add an irregular period, and you have the common symptoms of PCOS, a hormonal disorder that affects almost every tenth woman today.

It is the most common cause of infertility among young people, at least if they have someone with whom they want to have a child. The disorder seems to be a complication of metabolic syndrome. Abdominal obesity, elevated insulin levels, high blood pressures, and type 2 diabetes are common for PCOS. It sounds like one of the Western diseases.[22]

Today, these women aren't getting an effective treatment. What would happen if they tried a low-carbohydrate diet? It lowers the insulin and other abnormalities. What would

---

22. PCOS stands for polycystic ovarian syndrome. The ovaries have an abnormal number of follicles, as visible during an ultrasound. The disorder results in a surplus of testosterone, the male sex hormone. That disturbs the ovulation, which generates an irregular period and infertility. With time, it can produce more male hair growth, as with a teenage boy. For example, it can result in a mustache or strands of hair on the chin.

happen to the pimples, unwanted hair growth, and their periods? Two interesting studies have been conducted on this topic.

The first one studied ninety-six overweight women with PCOS and compared a diet with complex carbohydrates (lower GI) to other diets. The GI diet gave better results, with better regulation of the women's periods.

Only one smaller study has tested a stricter low-carbohydrate diet. Eleven overweight women with PCOS were advised to consume a maximum of twenty grams of carbohydrates per day for six months. Five women completed the regimen for the whole time period. They lost a lot of weight, improved their hormone levels, and two became pregnant during the study, despite previous infertility.

Those are great results, but the latter study is small and lacks a control group. It doesn't provide much evidence. What's even less scientifically impressive are the many positive reactions I have received via my blog, in the comments section, and emails from women who have tried it. Is there more?

In vitro or real food

I recently went on a cruise from Florida to the Bahamas. The boat housed hundreds of other low-carbohydrate enthusiasts, including a couple of doctors. One of them was Michael D. Fox (not the actor), a specialist on infertility.

Dr. Fox is tall, blonde, and notably thin for a middle-aged American. Perhaps because he barely eats a single carbohydrate. He is seemingly shy, but has spectacular stories to tell.

PCOS is extremely common in the United States, especially among infertile women. Dr. Fox talked about the transformation that took place when his fertility clinic started giving advice about a low-carbohydrate diet. Suddenly, infertile women could get pregnant without in vitro fertilization. As a bonus, they became thinner and healthier.

Dr. Fox is, like most Americans, very friendly. I wrote parts of this book with a view of the Atlantic Ocean, from the beach house that he lent me. He also showed me around his private practice in Jacksonville, Florida. The clinic was very exclusive, filled with antique furniture, but with a homey feeling. The examination rooms had names like "Lake Como" and "Tuscany," after his favorite places in Italy.

Dr. Fox worked in a white coat over green scrubs. His coat had a yellow mark with the text "Corn Syrup Kills," referring to the cheap sugar that almost all American industrial food contains. We know that sugar is bad, but did you know it could prevent you from having children? Two walls in the clinic are filled with photographs of newborn babies. Many of them were conceived after their mothers had stopped eating sugar-filled low-fat products. Dr. Fox himself has five children, of which three were triplets. He tries to keep them away from sugar and they are unusually healthy. But they don't avoid sugar entirely. Dr. Fox's wife is less convinced about the blessings of a strict low-carbohydrate diet. It's like they say: you never become a prophet in your own hometown.

But an increasing number of doctors see the correlation with fertility. In 2009, the Danish gynecologist Bjarne Stigsby wrote the book *Eat Yourself Pregnant*. He talks about how his patients often have such high insulin levels that it is the direct cause of infertility.

How do you eat yourself pregnant, according to Dr. Stigsby? Just like Dr. Fox, with a low-carbohydrate diet. That's to say, meat, fish, eggs, and vegetables. According to Stigsby, his patients often have normal periods and ovulation, which is conducive to a pregnancy.

Studies and reality show the same thing. There is an alternative to repeated expensive attempts with in vitro fertilization. Many women can eat themselves pregnant. They can eat themselves free of the hormone imbalance PCOS, one of the Western diseases.

Another Western disease predominantly affects men.

Male problems

Do you have difficulty peeing? Every third middle-aged man (or older) suffers from it. Their stream has become weaker with age. For many men, it is a disabling problem. It seems unreasonable that so many people are affected by it. In less developed countries, those issues used to be rare. If it is not a normal occurrence, what is the root cause?

The prostate gland can be found around the male urethra. In the Western world, it has a worrying tendency of growing with age. The problem is obvious. If the prostate grows too large, it tightens the urethra. It puts a stop to everything.

Associate Professor Jan Hammarsten specializes in prostate diseases and has long researched their root causes and the correlation with our lifestyle. He himself follows a paleo diet and avoids sugar and bread (for breakfast he often eats a boiled egg and mackerel in tomato sauce). He was very pleased with the results when I recently interviewed him.

About twenty years ago, Hammarsten noticed something that put him on an interesting research track. His patients with really large prostate glands were often obese and had diabetes. He suspected a correlation between prostate disease and metabolic syndrome.

After a couple of published studies, the picture is clearer. His suspicion was correct. Regardless of which part of metabolic syndrome Hammarsten's research group looked at—obesity, high blood pressure, or something else—it was a risk factor of an enlarged prostate. But one factor was stronger than all the others: insulin.

High insulin levels also generate higher production of the growth factor IGF-1 (Insulin Growth Factor). It can lead to increased cellular division and growth of many different bodily tissues. The more available growth stimulating hormone, the faster men's prostate glands seem to grow with time—and the more the gland tightens the urethra. It makes the urine stream shorter and shorter until it just falls straight down. In the end, they have to visit the bathroom more frequently, including at night.

Overweight patients are often recommended a low-carbohydrate diet by Hammarsten. Like other specialists, he often has short visits, but he usually discusses diets for three minutes and hands out a brochure with dietary advice. When I interviewed him, he ironically used advice from Dietdoctor.com. This quick intervention often resulted in his patients losing 22 lbs (10 kg). Hopefully their prostate shrinks a bit as well.

Hammarsten is convinced. An enlarged prostate is not a common side effect of aging. It is a disease that can be avoided. There are additional reasons for avoiding excess stimulation of the prostate's growth and cellular division. Perhaps you can already guess it. A high insulin level is also a heavy risk factor for death caused by prostate cancer.

Cancer—a Western disease?

Cancer diseases are, after cardiovascular disease, the group of diseases that now kill most Swedes. Cancer usually develops over a couple of decades when the cells in, for example, breasts, intestines, or lungs divide themselves uncontrollably. The culprit is harmful gene mutations in the genes that regulate cell growth. Growth factors in the body can perpetuate such cells and make the growth occur faster. In the end, the cancer can spread across the body and lead to death.

If there is a way of preventing or slowing down many cancer cases, it would be very meaningful. If the remedy was relatively simple, we would already know about it, unless, of course, if we have been looking in the wrong place.

Do you remember Albert Schweitzer, the missionary doctor who arrived in Africa in 1913 and later received the Nobel Peace Prize? Schweitzer was astonished during his first time there that he didn't discover a single case of cancer in the population. But during the following decades, more cancer cases started to arise simultaneously as the natives started eating like the white people.

There are several other similar cases. In a completely different environment, Eskimos traditionally subsisted on a very low-carbohydrate diet rich with meat. Dr. Samuel Hutton traveled to northern Canada and started treating them in 1902. He found that the Western diseases were notably rare. "The most striking thing is cancer," he noted after eleven years. "I have never heard of or seen a case of melanoma with an Eskimo."

In the book *Good Calories, Bad Calories*, science journalist Gary Taubes reviews twenty or so stories from doctors who worked in remote areas of the world during the early twentieth century. Back then, cancer was still a rare occurrence in many places. That is not true anymore.

The American statistician Fredrick Hoffman summarized several reports about the occurrence of cancer in different parts of the world during this period. In the book *Cancer and Diet* (1937), he concluded that the cancer mortality increased at a "more or less alarming rate around the world." This was sometimes increasing from a really low level: ". . . evidence shows that according to medically qualified observers, cancer is very rare amongst primitive populations."

Today, cancer is very common across the globe. What remains is the discrepancy between different *forms* of cancer in different countries. During the past couple of decades, several different reasons have been discussed. Of course, smoking (which, among many things, can cause lung cancer), various environmental toxins, viruses, genes, or simply age. If you discuss diet, the usual theory is bound to come up again.

A well-known dead end

If something in the diet causes cancer, saturated fat or meat was suspected for the past couple of decades. That is ironically what Dr. Samuel Hutton's patients largely subsisted on back in the day, when he claimed that cancer diseases barely existed among them. But we do not have to rely on such unwarranted stories. The theory has been tested in high-quality studies. Do you get less cancer from a low-fat diet?

In 2006, we found out the answer. That is when the largest (by far) study about the long-term effects of a low-fat diet was published. It was called Women's Health Initiative. Approximately fifty thousand women had been randomly selected into eating either low-fat or regular food for eight years. The low-fat diet failed miserably when it came down to cancer. The risk was not reduced, despite the participants eating more fruit and greens.

After that, the study examined three thousand women who had already had breast cancer. Half of them consumed less fat and more fruit, greens, and fibers. They were tracked for an average of seven years. The results were the same. Those who reduced their fat intake experienced the same number of cancer relapses and did not live longer.

A low-fat diet was not the answer. Fat didn't seem to pertain to cancer. It was time to keep searching.

Adding insult to injury

It is not just the increasing number of cancer diagnoses that speak to the fact that they belong to the Western diseases. It is also a fact that cancer has an evident correlation with other Western diseases.

Obese people have an increased risk of all sorts of cancer, such as breast, intestinal, esophagus, kidney, liver, and an increased risk of dying from prostate cancer. Type 2 diabetics also have an increased risk of other types of common cancers. Why?

There is a possible correlation between obesity, type 2 diabetes, and cancer. Growth factors. Obese people as well as type 2 diabetics typically suffer from high levels of the hormone insulin. That usually causes high levels of the growth factor IGH-1. Both insulin and IGF-1 stimulate cell partition. That might be crucial.

It is commonly accepted that cancer tumors start with a couple of independently unimportant mutations in your body's DNA. Such mutations disturb the otherwise meticulously regulated cell division, the first step toward a tumor. Fortunately, the road toward cancer is long. The mutated cell must continue to divide itself and to experience a couple of unfortunate divisions to become malignant. Even if you suffer from that bad luck, the process often takes decades or more.

You can compare little hints of starting tumors in the body with slowly glowing coal. With a little luck, it won't start a fire. Unless someone fuels it.

With high levels of the growth factor insulin and IGF-1, those cells get the signal to divide. Obese people and type 2 diabetics often have high levels of those growth hormones for part of their lives. It is bound to accelerate cancer growth. It is likely to increase the risk of cancer striking much earlier in life, such as at age sixty, instead of lying dormant until much later, perhaps until you have time to die of old age.

In the absence of proof

Even if the theory sounds plausible, more and more people are talking about how it was never tested in a large, high-quality study. They should return to do large, randomized intervention studies to find out if people actually get less cancer by eating a low-carbohydrate diet. Such studies haven't even begun.

Several studies have been conducted that focus on this area.

They have conducted several studies about low-fat diets: they do not prevent cancer. When it comes down to a low-carbohydrate diet, we don't know yet. But there are signs from observational studies that imply that the answer might be yes.

A study tracked 5,450 women over the course of eight years and several measurements of their insulin levels. When they compared the third of the women with the highest insulin to the third with the lowest level, it turned out that the women with high insulin had a 120 percent higher risk of breast cancer.

A study from the University of Umeå has examined data from half a million people from Sweden, Norway, and Austria. Those with elevated blood sugar had a distinctly increased risk of developing many types of cancer during the ten years they were tracked. The study is the largest of its kind in the Western world. An even larger Korean study showed similar results.

A lot of carbohydrates in your diet elevates the blood sugar and insulin, so what do studies reveal about people who eat a lot of carbohydrates? Two large reviews of all prior observational studies have been published in *American Journal of Clinical Nutrition* the last couple of years. They show that people who eat a lot of simple carbohydrates have a significantly higher risk of getting breast cancer, intestinal cancer, or cervical cancer.

Yet again—high-quality intervention studies have yet to be conducted. In conclusion, many types of cancer are significantly more common with obesity, type 2 diabetes, high insulin, high blood sugar, and high consumption of carbohydrates. There appears to be a clear correlation. And high levels of growth factors such as insulin can accelerate cancer development, like pouring gasoline on a fire.

Cancer was rare among primitive populations. Modern science is about to clarify things. Today, the most common forms of cancer seem to go together with the Western diseases. Other Western diseases have been shown to be suppressed by less sugar and flour in your diet. In theory it can also slow down the growth of cancerous tumors through reducing insulin and IGF-1.

Perhaps real food can even prevent cancer.

Your genes, your destiny

This chapter discussed how a simple change in your diet can have dramatic effects on your health. But the environment in which you live is only one of the two factors that impact your health. The other is, of course, your genes.

Are you doomed if you have a family history of Western diseases? Is it your destiny to get sick if you carry genes for obesity, cancer, or dementia? The short answer is no.

The common genes that increase the risk of, for example, type 2 diabetes, breast cancer, or Alzheimer's hardly determine your fate. They mean increased sensitivity. Back in the day, such genes were unlikely to result in severe disease. They would have been weeded out during evolution. Then they wouldn't have been so common.

Most likely these are about genes that make you extra sensitive to a new environment, one rich in sugar and starch.[23]

Some can eat more simple carbohydrates than others, without obvious harm. The world is unfair. But belonging to the sensitive group is not a reason to give up. Quite the opposite—it provides a reason to contemplate your lifestyle even more. It is then extra important for your health.

Avoid what you are sensitive to. At least then you can become just as healthy and thin as someone with fortunate genes. Of course nothing guarantees lifelong health, but you can significantly improve your chances.

Too good to be true?

You probably remember Weston A. Price from the first chapter, the dentist professor who traveled the world like Indiana Jones in the 1930s. He barely saw any cases where the new food didn't exist. The question was, if sugar and white flour can make teeth rot, what does it do to the rest of the body? We know that now.

Sugar and white flour seem to increase the risk for all the Western diseases, those which used to be rare but are now common. Here are a couple of good examples of Western diseases:

Obesity
Diabetes
Cardiovascular disease
Cancer

---

23. T. L. Cleave wrote eloquently about the difference between hereditary defects and hereditary characteristics in his book *The Saccharine Disease* in 1974. Many professors and experts need to read it today.

Cleave's more telling examples take place in the trenches of wwi. When infantrymen stormed the fortifications, tall soldiers were more often shot down by machine guns. Short soldiers had a better chance of survival.

No one would claim that the tall soldiers died from a genetic defect. Being taller could have been an advantage until the new environmental factor, the machine gun bullets, appeared. If tall people avoid things like that, they can do fine.

Dementia
Fatty liver
High blood pressure
Enlarged prostate
Sleep apnea syndrome
Gallstone
PCOS
Gout
Arthritis
Acne
Cavities
Osteoarthritis

There are more diseases that would probably fit into this chapter, diseases where more and more things show a correlation to the new food, which provides fascinating possibilities. But these will have to suffice for now while we await more knowledge on the area. The number of diseases can still be unreasonably large.

Less sugar and starch, is that the solution to everything? Can it make you thinner and protect against not just severe diseases, but also against acne, genital itchiness, and flatulence? Is it too good to be true? I don't believe so. This is what I think.

Avoid the new food so you can avoid the new diseases.

Starch-rich agricultural food is still pretty new. The Industrial Revolution's sugar and white flour is even newer. In the end, the fear of fat made us eat even more of the food we can't tolerate. That was the three-step process that caused today's epidemic of obesity, diabetes, and other Western diseases.

The food we handle the best should be what we have eaten the longest, that to which our bodies and genes have probably adjusted. You don't have to take my word for what type of food that was. Your ancestors showed it to us. They left messages, before anyone had invented agriculture.

A time window

We derive from the new humans, the Cro-Magnon people, who conquered Europe from the Neanderthals about thirty thousand years ago. They had many new characteristics that are familiar to us today. The new people did things that no one had previously done. For example, they painted. And many of the paintings still exist today.

We have found preserved paintings in caves in France, Spain, England, Finland, and Bulgaria. Search online for "cave paintings" and have a look. They are a window into a different world, the world from which you and I derive (Europe, tens of thousands of years prior to the development of agriculture). Our ancestors painted what was important to them and we can still see it.

The walls show wandering animals of prey: bison, oxen, and deer, sometimes followed by the humans hunting them. They are pictures from the world that we come from, pictures of the food for which we were designed.

And so, to the obvious—that which is *not* included in the painting. Colorful plastic casings with low-fat products, filled with starch and sugar, are nowhere to be found.

How could we ever believe that we need that for our health? What tricked us? Was there some truth in the last couple of decades' fear of fat and cholesterol?

Now it is time for the next piece of the world view puzzle. Now it is time to reveal the secret behind the biggest medical mistake in history. The reason behind a scary number of diseases across the world. Now it is time to kill the dragon.

CHAPTER EIGHT

Cholesterol: killing the dragon

Everyone I know in science—everyone—realizes that the simplified low-fat dietary advice was a mistake.

DR. RONALD KRAUSS
*Leading cholesterol researcher and one of the most prominent names behind
the American fat-fearing dietary advice.*

The fear of cholesterol is the foundation behind the theory about the dangers of fat. When the fear spread, the disaster sped up. Behind the fear of fat and cholesterol, the epidemics of obesity, diabetes, and other Western diseases have advanced across the world.

Now we realize the mistake. Low-fat diets were useless for health. But cholesterol correlates with heart disease. It just wasn't as simple as scientists thought in the 1950s or like commercials claim today.

Now it is time to reveal the truth. Today, the biggest strength of the fear of fat, the scary word cholesterol, could become its greatest weakness. It can mean more than tastier food. Perhaps it can save you and your family from disease and unnecessary lifelong medication.

Stay tuned for the details after the commercials.

"Hooligan behavior"

How do you get healthy people to eat industrial fat for health reasons? Perhaps by following the methods of the margarine brand Promise, which offers a free cholesterol test. Promise toured around grocery stores for a couple of years and let interested people test their cholesterol levels with a quick blood test.

If the number exceeded 200 MG/DL, the tested person was informed about the increased risk of heart attacks and how it could be reduced (first and foremost, by purchasing Promise's expensive and special margarine). It sounds like a good-hearted effort for public health. So why did the final tour end abruptly in November of 2008, after over a hundred stops in large grocery stores and tens of thousands of blood tests?

In a media scrutiny effort, a chief physician called their approach questionable and thought it was outrageous that no one had reacted earlier. Another doctor was upset that "objectively healthy people had become subjectively sick through their testing." A third doctor called it "hooligan behavior for scaring a bunch of predominantly older ladies."

After the media frenzy, Promise was blacklisted from the grocery stores in the next city, and that was the end of their cholesterol tours in Sweden. What was the problem?

Cholesterol-lowering margarine has never been proved to make anyone healthier. But that is not the main problem. The big problem is the obsolete term "high cholesterol." Does a cholesterol level above 200 mean that you risk having a heart attack and should avoid real food?

Every other healthy thirty-year-old person in Sweden has a cholesterol level above 5, and 95 percent of all sixty-year-olds do as well. But most of them do not have an abnormal risk of heart diseases. The cholesterol level says very little about a person's accumulated risk for disease. It is a very unsure and fuzzy metric. But it is lucrative if it can turn completely healthy people into scared customers.

When Promise had conducted the test, they were able to scare most customers with the fact that they risked dying from a heart attack since their cholesterol levels were above 200. Regardless of how healthy they were. Then they could sell them an expensive and chemical-filled margarine with no known health benefits.

You can see why it was called questionable and hooligan behavior.[24]

Promise's cholesterol tour is just a fun act. It is just a symptom of the mistake from the 1950s that happened to make hundreds of millions of people obese and sick. The fundamental mistake behind the entire fear of fat and the subsequent obesity epidemic.

The biggest medical mistake in history

The basis for the low-fat dietary ideology, from Ancel Keys's days, was the theory that *(saturated) fat raises cholesterol* and that *high cholesterol causes heart disease*. The message was clear: fat was dangerous.

Like we saw, the theory didn't work. Large, modern studies show no benefits from eating less fat, saturated fat, or cholesterol. Perhaps low-fat food is even dangerous for you.

Alas, saturated fat is completely harmless. But it can raise your cholesterol, at least a little bit, and in a short period of time. That is what got us lost. How does that fit together? How does the food you eat, the cholesterol, and the prevention of heart disease fit together? Ultimately, science can give us the answer.

The competition is fierce when it comes to dangerous medical mistakes. There are plenty to choose from. In the nineteenth century, medical students could go directly from the bodies in the autopsy room to examining pregnant women, without washing their hands. They didn't know what bacteria were or that it caused a horrifying number of women to die from postpartum infection.

Doctor Ignaz Semmelweiss proved that mandatory hand-washing saved a ton of lives in his delivery clinics. But his research was ignored for decades. New mothers kept dying from

---

24. To provide some context, I should also mention that Promise's margarine ads with questionable health arguments have recently been reported and convicted time after time. The Council of Market Ethics have convicted them for misleading advertising, they have received fines in Denmark for misleading advertising, and the Advertising Ombudsman has repeatedly found them guilty for illegal hidden advertising, e.g. paid advertising that has been created to look like unbiased information from journalists. It is difficult to dismiss all of this as single occurrences or mistakes.

dirty hands. Semmelweiss himself ended his days in a mental institution. We can learn from that story. Healthcare professionals should absorb new research, even when it is inconvenient.

Another big mistake was bloodletting. For two thousand years, until the nineteenth century, that was doctors' main treatment for all diseases. They drew patients' blood, often in large quantities, to "balance the bodily fluids." When the treatment was eventually examined, it was found to make patients sicker, not healthier. Yet doctors continued for decades, out of habit and conviction, to draw their patients' blood.

George Washington, the first president of the United States, had a bad cold on December 13, 1799. He had been out riding in the rain the day before. His ambitious doctors drew almost two liters of blood, about a third of his whole supply. George Washington died the next evening.

It is impossible to tell how many people died from bloodletting, but it is definitely many. Time after time throughout history, the same story emerges. Dangerous treatments that have been proven to have no effect live on as old habits.

A low-fat diet to "lower cholesterol" is our time's bloodletting. In 1984 when the fat and cholesterol phobia gained traction in the United States, around 13 percent of the population was fat. A generation later, that number has grown to 34 percent. The whole world has followed. The United States had exported its food culture (soda and French fries, sugar and starch), its fear of fat, and its obesity.

There are hundreds of millions of obese and diabetic people in the whole world, not to mention all other Western diseases. A disaster that is too large to understand, perhaps the biggest medical mistake ever. Or was it? Is cholesterol so harmful that it is worth it? What is cholesterol, really?

Essential for animals

Cholesterol is an essential building block in every cell in your body. Every cell membrane, the enclosing and protective shell of your cell, contains plenty of cholesterol that stabilizes the membrane. The heart in particular is built from plenty of cholesterol. It is a crucial substance for you.

What is more, cholesterol is also the building block for your steroid hormones, such as the sex hormones testosterone and estrogen. That might explain an involuntary side effect of cholesterol-reducing medications.

Cholesterol is an essential building block in every cell in all animals. That is why we talk about "animal" cholesterol-rich food, such as meat. It is usually perceived to be more dangerous to eat than leaves, nuts, and roots. That theory is pretty odd. Humans also belong to the animal kingdom. We are not plants. How can cholesterol be poisonous to consume when your own body is actually constructed from it? When your own body easily produces its own cholesterol? When people have always consumed food that contains cholesterol?

Our bodies usually adjust the production of cholesterol depending on need. If we eat a lot of cholesterol, less is produced. If we eat a little bit of cholesterol, our bodies produce more. In other words: eat all of the cholesterol-rich eggs you want, it is harmless.

But the body's regulation system for cholesterol can be disturbed. That is what is behind the misconception that cholesterol is dangerous. The reason for the dangerous disturbance has been found to actually be something other than what we once thought it was.

It is more complicated than they knew in the 1950s. All cholesterol is not bad. Low cholesterol is not necessarily better. The old picture is so simplified that it is meaningless. Modern science shows a more complex picture, which is better for your health.

Good cop, bad cop

The cholesterol in the blood is transported in two different types of packages, on their way to different areas in the body. There are two main packages that go in opposite directions. You have probably heard of them and been measured for them if you have measured your cholesterol: LDL and HDL. They are also called the bad and good cholesterol. Good cop, bad cop. It is still a Hollywood-esque simplification. But it is a step closer toward the truth.

What happens when you eat a lot of saturated fat? Your good HDL cholesterol rises. A high HDL is a statistically powerful protection against heart disease. This already disproves the theory that *fat raises cholesterol and causes heart disease.* Eating saturated fat and raising the HDL can give you higher cholesterol results, since HDL is a part of the cholesterol. But a high HDL means a lower risk for heart disease, not the other way around. Raising the correct cholesterol seems to be able to protect you against heart disease.

On to the "bad" cholesterol, LDL. Similar to a Hollywood movie, it has a more exciting role. Just like in movies, the evil LDL also has positive sides. Perhaps it is only the environment, his upbringing so to say, that led him to the dark side. Perhaps drugs? Too much sugar and starch, throughout a long period of time, can actually make LDL really evil.

LDL and HDL have opposite functions in the body. The good HDL transports excess cholesterol from the body to the liver for recycling. A lot of HDL appears to be about keeping things neat.

LDL packages have the opposite role; they transport cholesterol into the body. They are created in the liver like large LDL and then head into the bloodstream (the large LDL are called triglycerides, if you have a cholesterol test taken). The cells in your body can attract LDL and extract so much that the packages shrink. The cells can also absorb entire packages. Healthy people produce large packages that continue to shrink into average LDLs before they are absorbed. So far so good, it seems normal and harmless. The LDL transports the desired cholesterol, the building materials, out to your cells.

The problem is the Western disease. In afflicted people, the issue is that the cells no longer want to absorb entire LDL packages. They only absorb parts of them. The LDL keeps shrinking. The blood is therefore filled with small, dense LDLS. They may go rancid and appear to be able to harm and get stuck in the artery walls. They can be seen as abandoned packages that are littering. In the end, they risk clogging the arteries. These abandoned, small, dense LDLs seem to be the really dangerous, super-evil cholesterol. All cholesterol is not bad. Not even everything that is LDL cholesterol. The larger, "fluffier," normal LDL packages seem harmless.

Fat and saturated fat can raise an average-sized LDL, good cholesterol. They can easily be spotted, even in old tests. They used to think that they were the problem. That was the disastrous mistake. What they missed, what they couldn't see in older tests, were the small, dense LDL particles. The really dangerous ones. You're probably guessing how you get such villains into your blood.

A hint: not from eating fatty food.

How you can make 100 billion Swedish crowns

Promise's margarine money is small potatoes. The fear of cholesterol has made the pharmaceutical industry one of the most lucrative in the world.

The top-selling medication of all is Lipitor, from the company Pfizer.[25] It is one of the cholesterol-lowering drugs on the list of the top most lucrative medications. The pills called Lipitor gross over 10 billion dollars around the world per year.

The cholesterol-reducing Lipitor is a so-called statin. In Sweden, the most common form is called Simvastatin. Statins are the pharmaceutical industry's biggest modern triumph. They reduce the risk for heart attack and premature death amongst people with a heart condition.
So far, so good. Except for profit companies, which not only want to sell medication to those who have a demonstrated need for them. They want to sell as much as they possibly can.

On Pfizer's Swedish website www.kolesterol.nu, it says that everybody should have a cholesterol level below 5. Otherwise they

---

25. Pfizer is also the company behind the famous blue erection pill Viagra. But Viagra is listed far down on the list of the most profitable medication, around sixtieth or so. The medications at the top do not have an immediate positive effect. They are medications that should be taken daily, throughout life, to prevent disease. They often reduce the risk factors of metabolic syndrome. As you know, there is a way of doing so that has fewer side effects: eating real food, less sugar and starch. It should also prevent the need for blue pills.

can provide you with cholesterol-lowering medication via your doctor. With hundreds of billions of Swedish crowns, they can keep doctors informed with the help of an army of trusted pharmaceutical representatives.

Does that methodology sound familiar? Most healthy Swedes have a cholesterol level higher than 5, especially older people. Every third Swede is on cholesterol-reducing medication today. Suddenly the gigantic profits are no longer surprising. Like Aldous Huxley said: "Medical science has made such fantastic progress that there are barely any healthy people left."

So how do the enormously profitable statins that everybody seems to need actually work? How do they lower the cholesterol and how can they decrease the risk of heart disease? Turns out it is easier than you would think. Statins are an antidote.

Statins affect the enzyme in your cells, HMG-COA-reductase, or HMGR. Both names are abbreviations. If you think HMG-COA reductase sounds complicated, you should be happy that I am sparing you the entire name of the enzyme. It is three times as long and ten times as complicated. Please send your thoughts to all medical students who have to fill their brains with hundreds of similar chemical names and reactions. The risk is that they don't see the individual trees through the forest.

The enzyme HMGR can be called the cholesterol builder. It starts the production of cholesterol in your body's cells and determines how much of it should be produced. Statins get stuck in the HMGR and disturb its functionality. It is like throwing rocks at the body's cholesterol-producing machinery. Suddenly the body's cells have a difficult time producing their own cholesterol.

When the cells cannot build cholesterol of their own, they need to absorb more from the blood. The cells proceed to absorb more LDL packages. That can be a good thing for those with metabolic syndrome and an excess of abandoned, small, and dense LDL packages in the blood. The fact that statins also reduce the amount of cholesterol in the blood is probably an unnecessary side effect.

The reason that statins reduce the risk amongst people with a heart condition is probably that the small, dense, and dangerous LDL packages are eliminated.

So you could live as unhealthily as you want, eat junk food, and take a daily statin pill (and many other pills for risk factors), and then everything is well. Right?

The dark side of statins

Effective medications have side effects. That is also true when you sabotage the body's ability to produce cholesterol. The most common side effect of statins is light muscle aches and muscular weakness. That can make it difficult to stay in shape. How fun is it to train with tender and weak muscles? Fortunately, really severe cases, that is to say a life-threatening deterioration of the body's muscles, are extremely rare. But who wants to become weaker and be in pain?

The effect on one's sex life is another question mark. Cholesterol is, after all, the building block for our sex hormones. One study showed that there was an increased risk of impotence after consuming statins and there are plenty of case studies about people who become impotent from statins, and who regain their potency when they quit, and who (the really stubborn ones) become impotent when they take up the habit again.

Statins seem to cause memory loss and difficulty thinking clearly among some. That is not surprising, since the brain partially consists of cholesterol. Reduced mental capacity from statins, compared to placebos, even if subtle, has been demonstrated by a well-conducted study.

Alas, statins risk elevating your blood sugar, reducing your potency, and making you weak. If you have a heart condition and have a high risk of dying from a heart attack, the side effects might be worth the risk. But no one wants unnecessary side effects.

Is there no healthier way of preventing heart disease?

The poisoning and the antidote

So statins prevent the body from producing its own cholesterol by blocking the HMGR, the cells' cholesterol builders.

One might wonder if there is something that has the opposite effect, something that increases the activity among the HMGR. The answer to that question is yes. There actually exists such a thing, and it is familiar to you. The answer is insulin.

Suddenly the pieces of the puzzle are falling into place. Suddenly the image is a little clearer. The Western disease, metabolic syndrome, has had another manifestation. It is starting to become a well-known occurrence. A person with stone-age genes ends up in a new world filled with Coca-Cola and French fries, sugar and starch. The blood sugar spikes and so does the insulin hormone.

High insulin levels don't just mean you're storing a lot of fat. It also signals that the person has a nutritious diet and that it is time to create cholesterol. The HMGR enzyme gets to work. If it rarely happens, it might not be a problem. The problem will start to occur if you eat too much of such food repeatedly for a long period of time.

You could end up with constantly elevated insulin levels. You will develop metabolic syndrome. The HMGR is constantly activated. The cells produce plenty of cholesterol and you rarely need more. It therefore stops absorbing LDL packages from the blood. The blood is filled with undesirable leftovers, small, dense LDLs—those that seem to be harmful for the arteries and tend to accelerate the clogging. They are an additional consequence of the Western disease.

A sugar surplus via insulin could result in a harmful increase in the activity of the body's cholesterol-producing enzyme, that which statins prevent. The dangerous cholesterol disturbance seems to depend on sugar poisoning. The statins are an antidote.

Why not stop overdosing? Without poison you might not need the antidote.

The image becomes clear

Could it actually be sugar and not fat that provides a dangerous cholesterol disturbance? Does that have scientific evidence? The answer is yes. There is plenty of support. The simplified talk about "high cholesterol" falls flat in light of new knowledge.

Let us see how food really affects cholesterol. The following detailed image has been laid out by a leading cholesterol researcher and is becoming increasingly more accepted. See the reference chapter for more studies that go into it.

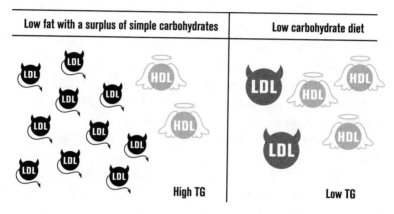

ON THE LEFT: *the metabolic hormone disturbance that means a high risk of heart disease: many small, dense LDLs that can get stuck in the arterial walls, fewer protective HDLs, and dangerously high triglycerides. The disturbance is caused by a carbohydrate surplus and is a part of the metabolic syndrome (along with abdominal obesity, high blood sugar, and high blood pressure).*

ON THE RIGHT: *a distribution with low risk of heart disease. Big, fluffy LDLs, low triglycerides, and many protective HDLs. This cholesterol distribution is produced by a low-carbohydrate diet. It can be the normal situation—when we eat that for which we are designed.*

Human studies show that the distribution of the cholesterol as shown above has a stronger correlation with heart disease than just cholesterol of the LDL value.[26] More details can be found in the reference chapter.

What does the new image mean for your health and our history?

The mistake behind the disaster

All the details mentioned above are new knowledge based on new research. Ancel Keys was not aware of any of it when he formulated the theory about the fear of fat in the 1950s. He simply knew that cholesterol seemed to be connected with heart disease in some way. He did not know the difference between LDL and HDL, and even less about the difference between different sized LDL.

It was here that the mistake arose. By eating less saturated fat, you can slightly lower your total cholesterol level. Keys thought that he had found the cure for heart disease. If people ate less saturated fat, their cholesterol would sink. In theory, it would save them from heart disease. We know that it failed. Now we know why.

What Keys didn't know was that the low-fat diet reduced the *good* cholesterol, HDL, which means an *increased* risk of heart disease. If the fat is replaced with carbohydrates, you also produce more of the dangerous cholesterol particles, the small and dense LDLs.[27]

---

26. The strongest risk factor in regular cholesterol tests is cholesterol/HDL. The cholesterol level divided by the HDL value. The lower the result, the lower the risk of heart disease.

If your cholesterol is 8 and your HDL is 2, the result is 4, pretty good. If your cholesterol level is reduced to 7 and your HDL is 1, the value is 7, not very good. A high cholesterol level can thus be better than a lower one. The same thing goes for LDL. The cholesterol level of LDL on their own are therefore very uncertain measurements.

Want to read more about risk evaluation of your cholesterol levels? Go to Dietdoctor.com/cholesterol—or search online for "cholesterol."

27. How does food with unsaturated fat really lower the cholesterol? That question seems difficult to answer. According to Ralf Sundberg, doctor and assistant professor with a special interest in the area, the following might be the cause:

The cell membranes should maintain proper consistency, not too solid and not too liquid. The more unsaturated fat you eat, the more saturated fat the cell membrane absorbs and they can become too liquidy. Then the cell increases the cholesterol in the membranes to keep the right consistency. But the cholesterol is absorbed from the blood until a new status quo is reached.

This ironic mistake could have been a funny detail in medical history. Instead it dragged the entire Western world into fearing fat and the ensuing misery.

Statins, which lower the LDL, protect against heart attacks among the already sick. That cemented the fear of fat. If a reduction of the LDL with statins helped, they believe that a reduction of the LDL using a low-fat diet would have the same results. That was not the case.

Now we know why. The positive effect of statins is most likely the reduced number of small and dense LDLs. The fact that they simultaneously reduce all the normal cholesterol seems to just be an unnecessary side effect.

Therefore, the obsolete cholesterol theory falls completely flat.

The death of the dragon

All cholesterol is not dangerous. It is an essential building block in all animals, including humans. All LDL cholesterol is not dangerous either. LDL is the cholesterol, the building blocks, that is transported out to the body's cells. It is a normal bodily function, just like the red blood cells that transport oxygen around your body.

We have been close to the truth, but we haven't seen it until now. The dangerous aspect is not the body's building block cholesterol or its normal transportation in the blood. The dangerous thing is the cholesterol disturbance included in metabolic syndrome, the Western disease. The imbalance that is associated with abdominal obesity, high triglycerides, and full of small, evil, and dense LDLs.

A low-fat diet with a surplus of insulin-increasing carbohydrates causes the dangerous cholesterol imbalance. Too much processed sugar doesn't only cause cavities, obesity, and diabetes. It also results in the cholesterol disturbance that is associated with heart disease. However, natural fat, including saturated fat, is harmless even for the cholesterol.

The mistake has been revealed. With a jujitsu throw, the last remaining triumph of the fat-fearing movement (i.e., cholesterol) is turned into another disadvantage. Then there are no remaining arguments. All important risk factors for Western diseases are naturally improved by a low-carbohydrate diet. They are all exacerbated by low-fat diet products. Even cholesterol.

The dragon is dead.

What does this mean for you?

Now you can eat tastier food with a clean conscience, and achieve better health with fewer medications. Eat all the natural fat you want, even saturated fat. Fry the food in butter if you want. It is not just tastier; it is good for your cholesterol.

At the same time as a low-carbohydrate diet improves your cholesterol, you get the other advantages that have been discussed. The risk factors for Western diseases are reduced. It gives you good chances for a healthier life.

Last but not least, you avoid having to unnecessarily take cholesterol-lowering pills or experimental specialty margarine. Most elderly Swedes have "high" cholesterol but could still have low risk for the diseases. They could be as healthy as could be. Still, they are often unnecessarily recommended lifelong medication with statins, a medication that can cause muscle ache and weakness, a medicine that increases the risk of diabetes, a medication from which many people fall ill.

A new review of all studies was published in 2010 in the renowned *Archives of Internal Medicine*. It examined whether there was proof of the benefit of statins for people without a known heart disease. The answer was, surprising for many, no. So there is no foundation for today's sprinkling of statins. There is no reason to start handing them out for free in McDonald's.

Statins, on the other hand, have a demonstrated effect on people with a heart condition. The reduction of heart disease could be worth the side effects, at least if you cannot achieve a perfect cholesterol distribution in any other way.

Here is this chapter's most important message: "High cholesterol" is not synonymous with risk of heart disease. If a large portion is the good HDL, it would actually be healthy. You need to take into account the distribution, otherwise you risk chewing statins for the rest of your life in vain.

Unfortunately not all doctors are aware of this yet. They have a lot on which to stay up to date. They don't have the same chance to read up on all new research that is being conducted. Please feel free to inform your doctor if he or she is still afraid of your cholesterol test, just because the result is above 200.[28] Perhaps you could pass this book on to your doctor when you have read it? Then you can help many patients that come after you.

A completely new worldview

Now we see the flaw in the theory about the dangers of fat: *saturated fat raises cholesterol* and *high cholesterol causes heart disease.* Researchers in the 1950s knew too little. Fat and saturated fat raises the good cholesterol. It statistically protects against heart disease. It is not fat, but sugar and starch, that produces the dangerous cholesterol, the small and dense LDL particles.

Evolution was right. Thomas Latimer Cleave and John Yudkin were right. But instead we tried, from the 1980s and onward, to do the complete opposite. The fear of natural fat had many people eating more sugar and quick carbohydrates. It created an epidemic of obesity and diabetes. Avoiding fat turns out to not be enough to help prevent heart disease. If anything, it increases the risk

---

28. Are you wondering what my cholesterol levels look like after years on a low-carbohydrate diet with all the butter and cream I have eaten? The answer is: excellent, thank you very much.

My latest cholesterol level was 209—average for a thirty-eight-year-old male. An entire 2.0 was in the form of HDL, uncommonly good for Swedish men. I attribute this to the tasty saturated fat. My cholesterol/HDL value is 2.7, indicating that I have a very low risk of developing heart disease.

A newer and more high-quality measurement for cholesterol is the apo ratio. It measures the number of LDL and HDL packages, instead of just measuring the volume. The lower the apo ratio, the lower the risk of heart disease. Most people fall under 1.5. The average for Swedish mean is around 0.9. Under 0.7 is very low and very good. I had 0.37—one of the best values I have ever seen. Even in studies, a low-carbohydrate diet produces the best apo ratio. Again, I must thank butter.

thereof. It doesn't even improve cholesterol. That was a mistake. Now we know and it is time to act.

It is time to throw out the failed fear of fat. Out with the industrially produced low-fat products. Out with the slightly hysterical cholesterol phobia that only benefits the pharmaceutical and margarine industries.

Bring back real food with natural ingredients. Food cooked with love and all the butter you want. From the ashes of the fear of fat, something new can take form. A completely new world view and a healthier future.

CHAPTER NINE

A healthier future

No army can withstand the strength of an idea whose time has come.

VICTOR HUGO

It is time for a health revolution. This final chapter pertains to how that can come about. How you can improve the world by first improving your health. How you can spread the message to those around you who are ready for it, those who want, and of course deserve, to know the way.

We have all the potential for great public health in Sweden. We are well off—we have food and a roof over our heads, clean water, airbags, universal healthcare, and antibiotics to fight infections. All these things have helped us live longer on average. What remains is to also live healthily, at least as long.

As a doctor, I see a lot of disease. A horrifyingly large part is today's Western diseases, chronic diseases that appear already in middle-aged people. We are used to it. But what if that isn't normal?

Imagine a country where heart disease is rare, where cancer is rare before old age. A country where we are thinner and healthy, filled with energy and a clean conscience despite eating our fill of real food. Where we happily move because it feels good, not because of being overweight. Where people even have calm stomachs, sleep well, more easily conceive children, and have good teeth. Where we are healthy up until old age, without the need for daily medication. A naturally healthy population.

It might be the future Sweden, a shiny role model for the rest of the world to imitate. It will hardly be easy, but we can reach the goal. You can help. We must spread the truth. It is far from impossible. Today, ideas spread faster than ever, and an idea whose time has come is unstoppable.

So what is the food revolution? How does it happen, and what can you do?

Eat real food

The revolution starts with you eating real food. Letting go of the obsolete fear of natural fat and cholesterol is the first step. That can sometimes be enough. There is no reason to be scared of eating meat, fish, butter, or eggs. That is excellent food, very nutritious and healthy. And it is tasty, too. The more of that type of food you eat, the more full you will feel. Then you don't have to eat as much bad food. Feel free to add above-ground vegetables for taste as much as you want.[29]

Step two is to remove unnecessary sugar. Almost all types of sugar are unnecessary; you don't need a single gram thereof. If you are already thin and healthy, this is often enough to make you feel better and make you stay healthy. If you have a couple of extra pounds, they usually disappear. And your teeth will thank you.

---

29. Above-ground vegetables are, of course, vegetables that grow above the ground. For example, cabbage, squash, cauliflower, broccoli, bell pepper, cucumber, spinach, mushroom, olives, or avocado. They contain very few carbohydrates, and those that exist are slowly and harmlessly absorbed by the body.

Root vegetables like potatoes (which grow below the ground) contain more starch. Be careful with those.

The last step, for those who suffer from weight issues, blood sugar problems, stomach-related issues, or who just want to try it out, is to reduce starch. When you eat more real food (step one) you will automatically eat less potatoes, pasta, rice, and bread, since you become fuller from the real food.

So the reduction kind of happens automatically. But you can benefit from intentionally eating as little starch-rich food as possible: find the level with which you are comfortable. Especially diabetics: if you want to lose weight or have a sweet tooth, you benefit from reducing the amount of starch. At first it is wise to avoid white flour, regular bread, and pasta. This chapter is followed by a beginner's guide with more detailed advice. There are also suggestions for breakfasts and other meals, recipes, a suggested grocery list, and so on. But it really isn't more difficult than what is mentioned above.

There are hundreds of reasons why it is worth trying. If you are hesitant, I suggest you give it two weeks. You can survive without sugar for two weeks, right? If you have a serious sweet tooth: congratulations, that is one of the best reasons for trying a low-carbohydrate diet. The desire often disappears in a couple of days when you stabilize your blood sugar and insulin. Bid the excess desire for sugar farewell and experience true satisfaction.

You can prove the effect on yourself. Natural fat doesn't make you fat, it makes you full. Enjoy eating tasty food until you are full, and still—unbelievable, but true—lose the extra pounds. In fair studies, a low-carbohydrate diet with unlimited quantities has been proven to have the best effect on weight at least ten times. But if you want to be convinced, try it for yourself.

Are you diabetic or do you happen to have a blood sugar meter? Then you can easily measure how stable your blood sugar becomes after following a low-carbohydrate diet (see chapter six). A stable blood sugar can produce a calmer temper. There are at least five randomized studies that were conducted on diabetics that show that they become healthier with fewer blood sugar-raising carbohydrates. Now if you still need to prove the earth is round— if you try it for yourself, you will know.

Do you have a difficult stomach with aches, gas, or perhaps diarrhea? A low-carbohydrate diet often has a quick, calming impact, especially if you avoid fiber-rich vegetables (fiber ferments to gas in the intestine). Again, try it, and you will see for yourself.

Are there any disadvantages? Well, it is true that you might experience some temporary discomforts, symptoms of sugar withdrawal. Some experience fatigue, dizziness, or nausea the first week. It usually passes fairly quickly, and there are some tricks to avoid such discomforts (see p. 199).

Once you pass the withdrawal symptoms, it is all downhill from there. Eat until you are satisfied with tasty food and become healthier and thinner. In the end, you might feel so good that your desire to exercise returns or increases. See it for yourself.[30]

Many often feel so satisfied that they want to make all their friends try it. But how does one accomplish that?

Be the positive example

How do you convince others to try what has worked for you? It might be easier and more painless than you think.

One thing is clear. Nothing makes people as curious as a positive example close by. If you become healthy, thin, and happy, your friends will want to find out exactly what you did. Your acquaintances will also want to ask you (those who don't have the guts will ask your friends instead).

If you try to convince people who aren't ready, they will be irritated. That is not necessary. When they are ready and curious, they will ask you.

Feel free to learn more so you can easily answer their questions. The fact that you have read this book is a great start. There is a FAQ in the back of the book if you are wondering about something in particular.

---

30. If you want to read stories from hundreds of people who have successfully tested a low-carbohydrate diet, go to www.Dietdoctor.com.

Perhaps your story will end up there in the future?

The most common question is whether or not it is indeed dangerous to eat real food, even if it makes you healthier and thinner. We are so brainwashed today that it might be difficult to let go of the fear of natural fat and cholesterol. Since they have always warned us about fatty food, it must be at least slightly dangerous, right?

The answer is no, it is completely harmless. It is as natural to eat fat with cholesterol as to drink water. Humans have always done it, for millions of years. Since the 1980s, we have been scared to death of real food, the same time the obesity epidemic started.

Modern scientific studies show the same thing. You don't become healthier from eating less fat; quite the opposite. Even if you consider all the studies about this topic, they show that those who eat the most saturated fat do not become sicker than others. Saturated fat is, after all, proven to be harmless. For the past fifty years, nothing we eat has been as meticulously scrutinized without evidence that is it harmful. Saturated fat (as in butter, eggs, fatty meat) is thus among the most harmless food you can get your hands on.

What about the cholesterol? Saturated fat might raise the good cholesterol, HDL. A high HDL equals a powerful protection against heart disease. So a low-carbohydrate diet results in good cholesterol levels. What causes the really dangerous cholesterol—small, dense LDL—is sugar and starch.

The last objection that needs to be addressed could be this: How do you know that, in the long run, it is good to eat less sugar and starch? Even if all health markers seem to quickly improve, even if people feel good, even if the clogging in the arteries decreases, could the opposite not occur after five, ten, or twenty years? Should we not wait for a couple of decade-long studies that will be conducted in the future? In other words, should we not wait an additional generation to correct our mistake?

No. Sure, it would be fantastic with big, perfect, and really long studies on low-carbohydrate food, those that cost tens of billions of dollars. I hope they will start soon. But we cannot wait for generations to see through the mistake of being scared of real food. We cannot blindly continue toward the dead end of the obesity and diabetes epidemics.

Seriously, avoiding the new food—the sugar and flour—how dangerous could it be? It is more reasonable to think the other way around. Since we do not have long-term studies that show that the new food is harmless, since everything points toward the opposite, we should be careful with it. That carefulness should include children, the elderly, pregnant and breastfeeding women, the sick, and the healthy—yes, everyone. People with excess weight, diabetes, and other Western diseases have the most to gain.

The point is that a natural low-carbohydrate diet isn't strange. It is just real food, the food we are designed to eat. The only reason it is perceived as odd is that we have gotten used to today's sugary, manufactured food. How can anyone perceive today's enormous amounts of soda and candy as normal[31], and instead think that meat, fish, eggs, and vegetables is an "extreme diet"? That unfortunately means they have lost track of reality. The only reason to call really traditional food "the fear diet" is that they have gotten used to the fear of fat and think it is normal. It is not; it is a sad parenthesis that lasted a couple of decades. It is a dangerous medical mistake, our modern version of bloodletting. Fortunately, its era is over.

Bring tasty lunches to work, and you will surely make everyone jealous, especially if they have brought low-nutrition premade food, or worse, if they are yo-yo dieting with low-calorie shakes. Give it some time, and they will start to ask you plenty of questions.

If you have time and feel like it, search local food producers. Try meat from grass-fed cattle, eggs from free-range chickens, newly caught fish, freshly cultivated vegetables, or mushrooms fried in butter. There is no better or tastier food.

---

31. According to a study conducted by the Swedish USDA, Swedish teenagers get 25 percent of their calories from soda, candy, ice cream, snacks, pastries, or desserts.

It might take some time to digest it all. Feel free to discuss with others who are interested, read and learn more. The more you learn, the easier it will be for you to spread the knowledge to those around you who ask and need to know.

That is how the revolution starts. No one can force you or your friends to eat food that you do not want. No one can make you purchase it. When fewer and fewer want the manufactured fake food with its weird ingredients, it remains on the shelves, with more desperate special prices. We already see signs of it.

We need more real food in the future. Locally produced food can become more popular and in demand, to the joy of all local food producers.[32]

It could lead to lots of new job opportunities. The number of farmers in Sweden is only a fraction of what it used to be. Perhaps it is time to turn around the development? Producing quality food might be a future job again. Swedish food culture might be making its return.

A transformed production is an evident consequence of a change in demand. Those who want to preserve the status quo will claim that it is impossible. But we have solved bigger problems than that. Every time you shop in the grocery store, you choose what you want to support. Coca-Cola and Unilever, or local farmers? You have the power.

Soon the producers of disease-inducing fake food filled with sugar and additives might need to use their factories for something else. At the same time, we eat more natural food and are healthier than ever. That is how the revolution takes place, from the bottom up. Then only one thing remains.

---

32. Of course the food production must also be environmentally friendly. Hopefully the debate can leave behind the black and white idea that animal farming is always dangerous and vegetarianism is always good for the environment. Oranges and bananas from the other side of the world that are consumed in Sweden all year round are an environmental disaster. Cultivating grains with the help of artificial manure created from fossil fuels isn't good either. However, animals that are kept free and grazing create a continuously thicker earth layer.

The environmental issue is complicated. It deserves more contemplation than the over-simplified arguments.

Show them reality

What if more doctors, nurses, dieticians, and diet directors in municipalities and regional departments would learn more about low-carbohydrate food and health? It is happening slowly but surely. What if it wouldn't take centuries (like bloodletting) or decades (like hand-washing), but only a couple of years? Or at least only a decade? That would be fantastic.

That would accelerate the development toward a healthier population. At the same time, they would have the pleasure of seeing their patients healthier and thinner. Instead of requiring more medication with age, many patients would need less. Believe me, that is a delight to see.

There is an effective way to affect healthcare professionals. Show them reality. Doctors believe their own eyes. Even dieticians can do that in the end.

Doctors are better at switching paths than dietitians and others with dietary training. Doctors only studied nutrition for a couple of weeks during their core curriculum, while they were informed of medications and surgeries for years. Therefore they are not as stuck in the old fear of fat theory.

At the same time they are used to medical progress going forward and old methods becoming obsolete. Many know of the proverb "half of medical knowledge is incorrect, the problem is that you don't know which half." The theory about the dangers of fat has become obsolete and doctors rarely have a difficult time absorbing this.

It is simple to convince a doctor. It can be enough to have a couple of patients that test it and get spectacular health benefits. If they tell you how they did it, the doctors will automatically be curious, and if he or she starts to read the studies, then 1+1 could quickly add up to 2. So if you have gotten great health results from a low-carbohydrate diet, please tell your healthcare staff. That way you can speed up the paradigm shift, and you can help hundreds of patients who follow you.

Do you remember Dr. Eric Westman, the doctor who plays the piano for patients when they have lost weight? He was as skeptical as other people in the 1990s. After having seen his patients lose weight and become healthy due to the Atkins diet, he started reading up on the matter. Now he is conducting research and working exclusively with low-carbohydrate diets.

Not even the biggest skeptic, a doctor who a couple of years ago warned about low-carbohydrate diets in the *Doctor's Magazine* and now *DN Debatt*, is immune to persuasion. In a recent interview he said that a low-carbohydrate diet might be a good diet for severely overweight people. "For some," he said, "it has really been a success story." It is very impressive that he is nuancing himself from the original standpoint.

Most people eventually believe what their eyes show them. So let healthcare personnel know what you eat.[33]

Do you want to do more? Give this book to your doctor once you finish it. The chapter regarding cholesterol will be particularly useful. Doctors fear cholesterol. They need to learn the difference between the simplified term "good cholesterol" and a dangerous disturbance of the cholesterol due to too much sugar and starch. Then they can be ready to see things clearly. Then they can be ready to help their patients more than ever before.

What I discuss above is what causes a slow but steady revolution, step by step. Perhaps you are one of those who aren't going to wait?

A bonus for rebels

Do you want more? Perhaps you don't settle for being a positive role model and waiting for the world to change. Are you too angry because you yourself or your loved ones have become unnecessarily sick? Do you, like Charlie Abraham's dad, the guy behind The Charlie Foundation, feel like something needs to be

---

33. One last example is Dr. Thomas Bolte. He worked at Dr. Robert Atkins's clinic during the 1990s. But he hesitated to take the job. During the interview he asked: "But I don't believe in a low-carbohydrate diet!" Atkins laughed and answered: "Don't worry. You will."

With time, Dr. Bolte saw many obese type 2 diabetics become healthy almost miraculously. Other doctors keep asking him, a decade later, if he believes in a low-carbohydrate diet. His answer is usually: "Like I believe in oxygen."

done right away or preferably yesterday? Do you want to speed up the process?

Perhaps you have an ace up your sleeve. Perhaps you have your own idea about how things could change. Try it and please post to Dietdoctor.com if you succeed.

You might even replicate Jim Abraham's idea. Spreading the knowledge about the effects of low-carbohydrate food on pediatric epilepsy resulted in parents everywhere demanding the same help for their children. Soon, numerous hospitals offered that alternative.

Perhaps something similar could take place in Sweden. Many well-conducted studies have demonstrated that a low-carbohydrate diet has the best effect on obesity and diabetes. As a result, the new Swedish patient safety law now entitles you to receive help with a low-carbohydrate diet from the healthcare industry. You don't just have a moral right to it; even the law is on your side. Are you ready for battle? Help others by claiming your right. When more people do it, the healthcare industry is required to adjust.[34]

Those of you who work in the healthcare system don't have to wait for patients to demand the best advice. You start offering them today. Since the National Board of Health and Welfare declared in 2008 that a low-carbohydrate diet accords with science and tested experience, you can relax. Information materials for yourself or patients are available at www.Dietdoctor.com.

Dietitians and diabetes nurses in particular have much to gain from updating their recommendations. If you spend time on dietary recommendations, why not maximize the effect? Your job will become more fun if the patients are happier and healthier.

----

34. Patient Safety Law (2010:659) chapter 6. Obligations of the healthcare and hospital industry, et. al. 7 §: "When there exist several treatment alternatives that accord with science and tested experience, those who have the responsibility for the health of an individual must ensure that the patient is given the opportunity to choose the alternative that he or she prefers." The same requirements exist for counties (3 a §) and municipalities (18 a §) in the healthcare and hospital law.

Links to appropriate studies (as well as their conclusions) for print and use when needed are available at www.Dietdoctor.com/vetenskap.

That means professions like yours will become even more important in the healthcare industry.

The free brochures with dietary advice about blood sugar-raising carbohydrates from companies that sell blood sugar-reducing medication, you could preferably burn. If you receive one of them, why not protest?

One thing is worse than those brochures. That is when your tax money is used the same way.

The last obstacle

There is one development obstacle in Sweden: the Swedish USDA (SLV) and its attempt to stick to the low-fat dietary advice. Modern science shows that naturally saturated fat is harmless, in sharp contrast to what SLV has always claimed. Its latest statement? Even if it is harmless, it is *still* important to "substitute it" for artificial low-fat margarine. The logic is becoming unfathomable. Perhaps it is more about stubbornness and fear of losing.[35]

Healthy adults can ignore them and their keyhole markings. Many already do. But the SLV decides the food that is served in schools, hospitals, retirement homes, and some restaurants in Sweden. Those who eat there cannot escape. Many dietitians and dietary executives still take the advice of SLV very seriously.

Does that sound like an unimportant detail? Then think about this. Diabetics in hospitals and retirement homes have to settle for sugary juice, low-fat milk, and dry bread as breakfast or a snack. Food that could effectively spike their blood sugar and make them sicker. Low-fat products are everywhere. The meals are not necessarily better.

---

35. Despite the absence of scientific support, they still advise Swedes to follow a low-carbohydrate diet, with a higher part sugar and starch, just like they have been doing since the obesity epidemic started in the 1980s. In practice, they have simply copied the American dietary advice (which is now the world's most obese country). A wise idea?

More about SLV's evasive claims about "fat changes" in the Q&A section.

Several hospitals serve their patients with the scandalous food: plastic-wrapped and reheated boxes with additive-rich content. Starch is cheap, so the manufacturer Sodexo probably doesn't have an issue following the recommendations of SLV. But that doesn't make it real food. According to some, it is barely edible (54 percent of the patients are dissatisfied, according to one evaluation).

The dietary advice for children is an additional problem. According to the dietary advice of SLV, all children should eat key-hole-marked low-fat food. For example, "all children, despite age or weight" are advised to consume only a low-fat diet after they stop breastfeeding. According to SLV, any milk above 0.5 percent fat is considered dangerous for children and their cholesterol levels. Interestingly, breast milk contains about 4.5 percent fat, of which a large chunk is saturated. No one has probably thought of that. No one would think breastfeeding mothers are poisoning their children, right?

School children who only receive low-fat products feel less full. They become hungrier and more tired in class, and easily run across the street to purchase sweet energy drinks like Burn, Monster, or Red Bull to elevate their energy. Instead, the Swedish USDA should protect children from unnecessary amounts of soda, candy, and chips, rather than unnecessarily stop them from eating real food.

What can you do about it? Please feel free to protest. Make sure that they at least have filling, normal alternatives for those who want it. Dietary executives can follow their conscience. They do not need to follow obsolete advice that might be harmful to children, sick people, and others. Many have already started. Yet again, the revolution takes place from the bottom up.

They react very slowly at the top. Like Professor Martin Ingvar wrote about today's dietary advice in his new book *Hjärnkoll pa vikten*: "It seems like they are reluctant backing into the future." The SLV's foundational dietary advice is only updated once a decade, the last of which took place in 2004. It is of course unreasonable to wait years to correct a mistake or even admit to one. If the

Swedish USDA wants to do the right thing and maintain the public's trust, it is time to act now. It would nice if they didn't need the media's attention first.

It is not easy to admit old mistakes. It is difficult. But to do it, to correct them, is honorable. It is worth some respect. Perhaps we can all keep that in mind.

We actually have some exciting times to look forward to. Regardless, when the brake is released, the development is making progress. Modern science and regular people's experience all pull in the same direction. This section of the book was a bonus to those who want to do something extra. Perhaps you don't feel that way. Perhaps you just want to eat tasty food, keep healthy, and feel good. There is nothing wrong with that. Quite the opposite. It can get you far.

Forward

It starts with you. You can change your surroundings. It is revolutionary to try it for yourself and learn more. The book ends with a section of tips for beginners and where to find more information if you are interested. Try it and let the effect on your own health and weight make you happy and convince you. Release yourself from discredited theories and get a more modern view on food and health. Then tell your friends if they are interested, especially those with weight problems and diabetes. Please give this book to a friend when you have finished reading it.

When others make the same journey and spread the knowledge more broadly, more and more people will know more quickly. It will become impossible to stop. One person cannot change the world. But a million people can.

III.

Guide

CHAPTER TEN

The Enjoyment Method / LCHF for beginners

> **PLEASE EAT:**
> *Meat, fish, eggs, above-ground vegetables,*
> *and natural fat (like butter)*
>
> **PREFERABLY AVOID:**
> *Sugar and starch-rich foods*
> *(e.g. bread, pasta, rice, potatoes)*

Eat real food when you are hungry, until you are full. It is as simple as that. Let's see what this means in practice.

Real food

Real food is similar to that which humans have consumed for millions of years, the food for which our bodies are designed. Unfortunately there are plenty of cheap imitations in stores today. Fake food that is so unnatural that it cannot even go bad—not even microorganisms can survive off of it. Here are three fundamental pieces of advice to avoid fake food:

1. Avoid products that are filled with strange ingredients with names that you can barely pronounce. Not because they are necessarily harmful, but because that is only required in fake food.

2. Avoid too much sugar or starch (often the same products as bullet number 1)

3. Avoid diet products (often the same products as bullet numbers 1 and 2)

Western junk food is often guilty of violating at least two of the above rules. Avoid it and you have taken a big step toward better health. More detailed advice follows here:

DIETARY ADVICE

Please eat

MEAT: Any kind. Beef, pork, game, poultry. The fatty part is healthy as well as the skin of the chicken. Preferably choose organic and grass-fed meat.

FISH AND SEAFOOD: All types. Preferably fatty fish like salmon, mackerel, or herring. Avoid breading.

EGGS: In all forms. Boiled, cooked, omelet. Preferably organic.

NATURAL FAT, FATTY SAUCES: Feel free to use butter and cream in your cooking, and it will become tastier and you will feel fuller. Béarnaise sauce, hollandaise—read the labels or make your own from scratch. Coconut fat, olive oil, and canola oil are also good alternatives.

ABOVE-GROUND VEGETABLES: All types such as cauliflower, cabbage, Brussels sprouts, asparagus, broccoli, squash, eggplant, olives, spinach, mushrooms, cucumber, lettuce, avocado, onions, bell pepper, tomatoes, etc.

DAIRY PRODUCTS: Always choose the highest fat content. Plenty of butter, cream (40 percent), sour cream, fatty cheeses. Full-fat Greek/

Turkish yogurt. Be careful with regular milk and yogurt—they contain a lot of dairy sugar. Avoid flavored, sugary, and low-fat alternatives.

NUTS: Great as a TV snack (preferably in reasonable amounts).

BERRIES: Okay in reasonable amounts, unless you are super strict or sensitive. Great alongside whipped cream.

Preferably avoid

SUGAR: Worst of them all. Soda, candy, juice, sports drinks, chocolate, cookies, rolls, pastries, ice cream, breakfast cereals.

STARCH: Bread, pasta, rice, potatoes, French fries, chips, porridge, granola, and so on. "Whole grain products" are just a little less bad. Reasonable amounts of root vegetables are okay if you are not meticulous about the carbohydrates.

MARGARINE: Industrial butter imitations with an unnecessarily high omega-6 content. It provides no health benefits and tastes bad. It is statistically linked with asthma, allergies, and other inflammatory diseases.

BEER: Liquid bread. Unfortunately filled with malt sugar.

FRUIT: A lot of sugar. Could occasionally be consumed as candy.

Reward yourself at parties

You decide when it is party time. Your weight loss might slow down a bit.

ALCOHOL: Dry wine (regular red wine or dry white wine), whisky, brandy, drinks without sugar.

DARK CHOCOLATE: At least 70 percent cacao, preferably just a small piece.

Drinks during the week

WATER: Flavored or carbonated if you need it.

COFFEE: Preferably with heavy cream—try it!

TEA: Black, green, white . . .

THEORY

Warnings for diabetics

Are you diabetic? A strict low-carbohydrate diet might quickly make you too healthy for your medications. Be extra careful with insulin injections; your blood sugar may fall too low if you overdose. Many diabetics need to immediately reduce their insulin dosage by around 30 percent or more when they avoid carbohydrates. Those of you who are only treated with metformin pills do not risk plummeting blood sugar levels.

Meticulously regulate your blood sugar and adjust the medication accordingly in collaboration with your doctor and diabetes nurse if possible. If you are unsure how to adjust your medication according to your blood sugar, you must seek advice.

Hormonal weight regulation

Carbohydrates, simple as well as complex ones, all break down in the stomach to simple sugars. The sugar is quickly absorbed in the blood and raises the blood sugar, which increase the production of the hormone called insulin. That is the body's fat-storing hormone.

In large amounts, insulin prevents the burning of fat and stores the nutritious excess in the fat cells. A couple of hours after a meal it might result in a nutritional deficit in the blood, which creates a feeling of hunger and a sweet tooth. That easily translates into one eating more, preferably carbohydrates, which could lead to a vicious cycle of weight gain.

On the contrary, a low intake of carbohydrates results in a lower and more stable blood sugar level and thus a lower insulin level. That increases the burning of fat from the fat tissue and increases the fat metabolism. As a consequence, the body fat usually successively decreases, especially in people who suffer from abdominal obesity.

The intake of calories usually spontaneously decreases in studies when trial participants eat until they are full from a low-carbohydrate diet instead of a carbohydrate-rich diet. Alas, no counting or weighing is necessary. Thus, you can forget about calories and trust your hunger or feelings of satiation. Most people don't have to count or weigh their food more than they need to count their breaths. If you don't believe me, try it for a couple of weeks and see for yourself.

No animals in nature need the help of nutritional experts or calorie charts in order to eat. If they just eat the food for which they are designed, they will stay thin and avoid cavities, diabetes, and heart disease. Why would humans be any different? Why would you be different? Avoid the new food. With a little luck, that might be enough to keep you healthy and thin.

Studies don't just prove that your weight improves with a low-carbohydrate diet, but also your blood pressure, blood sugar, and cholesterol level. A calmer stomach and reduced sweet tooth are also common experiences.

Withdrawal symptoms

If you abruptly stop eating sugar and starch, you might experience withdrawal symptoms for the first week. You can equate it to "sugar withdrawal." For most people, it is endurable and passes quickly. Otherwise, there are ways of reducing the symptoms.

Headaches, fatigue, dizziness, minor heart palpitations, and irritability are common during the first couple of days. These symptoms will quickly pass once the body gets used to them. The issues can partly be avoided with additional fluids and salt throughout the first week. A good way might be a (sugar-free) cube of boullion in a mug with hot water from time to time, for example every fourth hour. Alternatively, you could drink a couple of extra glasses of water per day or add some salt to your food.

The reason is that a carbohydrate-rich diet binds water in the body and makes you more bloated. If you reduce that type of food, you will lose liquid through the kidneys. It may cause dehydration and sodium deficiency for the first week before your body gets used to it, which might result in a headache, dizziness, etc.

Some people prefer to slowly wean themselves off of carbohydrates to reduce the worst kind of adjustment issues. But for most people, the best thing is to go cold turkey. Some people lose excess water weight immediately during the first couple of days in order to keep up motivation.

Few carbohydrates

The fewer carbohydrates you eat, the more evident the effect on your weight and blood sugar will be. I recommend that you strictly follow the weight and blood sugar with which you are comfortable and happy. When you are satisfied with your weight and healthy, you might gradually try to eat more liberally.

Additional questions?

If you are confused about anything, the next chapter is filled with questions and answers about a low-carbohydrate diet. Before then, here are some dietary tips.

TIPS AND RECIPES

Breakfast suggestions

Egg and bacon
Greek yogurt with linseeds, sunflower seeds
Omelet
Yesterday's leftovers
Coffee with cream
A can of mackerel and boiled egg
Boiled egg with mayonnaise or butter
Avocado, gravlax (cured salmon), and sour cream
Sandwich with *oopsie bread* (see p. 205)
A piece of cheese with butter

Boiled egg mashed with butter, chopped chive, salt, and pepper
A piece of brie with ham or salami

Lunch and dinner

Choose meat, fish, or chicken dishes with vegetables and a fatty sauce. There are many alternatives to potatoes, such as mashed cauliflower (see p. 206). Drink water, or a couple of glasses of wine if it is a more festive occasion. There are more tips among the recipes if you continue reading.

Snacks/ if you want to eat something

When you follow a low-carbohydrate diet with more fat and protein you often stay full longer. Do not be surprised if you no longer need to snack. Many people subsist off of two or three meals a day. Here are some tips if you feel like snacking:

Rolled up ham or cheese with vegetables (tough guys spread butter on top)
Olives
Nuts
A piece of cheese
A boiled egg
A can of mackerel in tomato sauce

Olives and nuts can replace chips in front of the television. If you always feel like snacking in between meals, you are probably eating too little fat. Don't be afraid of fat. Eat more fat until you feel full.

Eating out/ at dinner parties

It usually works well to eat out. You can ask them to switch out the potatoes for a salad. Request extra butter with meat dishes so that you become full.

As far as fast food goes, the hamburger is often the least bad thing— of course you should avoid the soda and fries; drink water. Max (a Swedish burger joint) has low-carb burgers without bread that are served in a piece of lettuce. Pizza toppings are usually okay to eat, but the stricter you are, the more you need to avoid the pizza bread and edges.

If you are stricter with your diet during the week, it is easier to make exceptions when you are a guest at a dinner party. If you are unsure of what you will be served, you can eat yourself half-full at home before.

Plastic-wrapped Babybel cheese or a bag of nuts are popular as emergency snacks.

Grocery list for beginners

Butter
Heavy cream (40 percent)
Sour cream (34 percent)
Eggs
Bacon
Meat (minced, steak, pork chop, filet, etc.)
Fish (the fatty kind such as salmon or mackerel)
Cheese (full fat)
Greek yogurt
Cabbage (cauliflower, Brussels sprouts, etc.)
Above-ground vegetables
Frozen vegetables (broccoli, wok vegetables, etc.)
Avocado
Olives
Olive oil
Nuts

Clean out the pantry

Do you want to maximize your chances of success? Especially if you have a difficult sweet tooth or sugar addiction, you will benefit from cleaning out or throwing away (or donating) sugar- and starch-rich food, low-fat products, and similar foods:

Candy
Chips
Soda and juice
Margarine
Sugar of all sorts
Flour
Pasta
Rice
Potatoes
Everything that says "low fat"
Frozen dinners
Ice cream
Cookies

The snake in paradise

Be very skeptical of certain "low-carb" products such as pasta or chocolate. Unfortunately they work poorly and have disrupted many people's weight-loss attempts. They are usually filled with carbohydrates when you see through their creative marketing efforts.

For example, Dreamfield's "low-carbohydrate pasta" almost only consists of carbohydrates that are absorbed effectively by the body, albeit slowly. The low-carbohydrate chocolate is usually filled with sugar alcohols, which the sales representatives don't count as carbohydrates. Around half of them can be absorbed by the body and raise the blood sugar. The rest end up in the large intestine and create gas and diarrhea. Of course they also stimulate one's sweet tooth.

If you want to become healthy and thin, you should eat real food instead.

RECIPE IDEAS

At Dietdoctor.com there are links to thousands of free recipes and menus as well as printable advice that fit on the refrigerator.

Visit dietdoctor.com/low-carb/recipes for delicious low-carb recipes and meal plans.

There are already tons of cookbooks that focus on low-carbohydrate diets/LCHF. You will find some of them in any bookstore.

Additionally, you can often use recipes from cookbooks that focus on GI (glycemic index) or regular cookbooks by reducing the amount of carbohydrate-rich ingredients and slightly increasing the volume of fat.

Egg recipes

SIMPLE, WITH ONE EGG

Option 1: Place the egg in cold water and boil for four minutes to make a soft-boiled egg, or eight minutes for a hard-boiled egg. Enjoy it with some mayonnaise or butter.

Option 2: Fry it in a couple of tablespoons of butter, on one or both sides. Season with salt and white pepper.

Option 3: Melt some butter in a frying pan and add two eggs and two to three tablespoons of heavy cream per portion. Season with salt and pepper to taste. Stir the scramble continuously until it solidifies as much as you want. Feel free to add a couple of tablespoons of chopped chives and garnish with grated cheese. Serve with fried bacon.

Option 4: Make an omelet with three eggs and two tablespoons of heavy cream with salt and spices (white or black pepper, or anything else). Melt butter in a frying pan and add the batter; do not keep the heat too high. When the omelet has solidified on the surface, you can fill it with something tasty. For example, one or two types of cheese, fried bacon, mushrooms, good sausage (read the nutrition label), or leftovers from last night's dinner. Fold the omelet in half and serve with a crispy salad.

Instead of bread

Do you have a difficult time living without bread? Oopsies are a good alternative. It is similar to "bread" without carbohydrates, which can be consumed in many different ways.

Oopsie bread

This recipe yields six to eight pieces, depending on how big you make them:

3 eggs
3.5 oz (100 g) cream cheese
A pinch of salt
Half a tablespoon psyllium husk (may be excluded)
Half a teaspoon of baking powder (may be excluded)

Crack the eggs and separate the yolks from the whites. Whisk the whites to a hard foam along with the salt. You should be able to turn the bowl upside-down without pouring anything out. Then whisk the yolks and the cheese to a smooth batter and add the psyllium husk and baking powder if you want; that is what makes the oopsie more bread-like. Carefully fold the egg whites into the yolk batter to preserve the air in the whites. Place six to eight small spoonfuls of oopsie batter on the baking sheet and bake in the middle of the oven at 300 degrees Fahrenheit (150 degrees Celsius) for about twenty-five minutes until they turn a nice color.

They can be consumed as a sandwich or be used as hot dog or hamburger bread. You can also sprinkle them with different types of seeds before baking them, such as poppy seeds, sesame seeds, or sunflower seeds.

You can also make one large oopsie that can be used as the base for a Swiss roll. Just add a couple of layers of heavy cream (why not add some vanilla extract?) and your berries of choice.

Instead of potatoes

MASHED CAULIFLOWER: Split the cauliflower into smaller florets and boil them with salted water that you then pour out. Add cream and butter until you achieve the right flavor and texture and then mash with a mixer.

SALAD made from above-ground vegetables, preferably with different types of cheese. Try different kinds!

BOILED BROCCOLI, cauliflower, or Brussels sprouts.

CHEESE BAKED VEGETABLES: Fry, for example, squash, eggplant, fennel, or other vegetables that you like in butter and add salt and pepper. Place in an oven dish and sprinkle grated cheese on top, bake at 450 degrees Fahrenheit (225 degrees Celsius) until the cheese has melted and turned a nice color.

CREAMED VEGETABLES, such as green cabbage or spinach.

CAULIFLOWER RICE: Shredded cauliflower that is boiled in salted water for a couple of minutes provides a good alternative to rice.

AVOCADO

DELICIOUS DIPS, such as egg and shrimp mix. Hard-boil and chop a couple of eggs, peel one or two handfuls of shrimp, finely chop a small red onion. Mix equal parts sour cream and mayonnaise and add the eggs, shrimp, onion, chopped dill, and some caviar.

The alternatives above go well with meat, fish, and chicken instead of potatoes, pasta, rice, bulgur, etc.

Snacks and desserts

MIXED NUTS

SAUSAGE WITH A HIGH CONTENT OF MEAT AND FAT: Cut into small pieces; cut an equally sized cube of cheese and join with a tooth pick.

VEGETABLES WITH DIP: Cucumber sticks, pieces of bell pepper, cauliflower.

CREAM CHEESE ROLLS: Roll up a piece of cream cheese of any kind in, for example, a slice of salami, dried ham, or thinly-grated cucumber slices

OLIVES: Feel free to marinate them yourself. Add tasty olive oil and chop and add in basil, oregano, and a clove of garlic. You may also use dried spices.

LCHF CHIPS: Shred Parmesan (or another hard cheese that you like) and place small piles on a baking sheet, place in the oven at 450 degrees Fahrenheit (225 degrees Celsius), let them melt and get a nice color, then take them out and serve as chips. Feel free to serve with a good dip. Do not leave them in the oven without sporadically checking, as they easily burn.

Pancakes made with almond flour

Almond flour can be ordered online or purchased in most grocery stores; it consists of finely ground almonds that contain a low volume of carbohydrates. Of course, you can also make it yourself in a food processor.

4 eggs
⅓ cup (300 ml) heavy cream (40 percent)
⅖ cup (200 ml) almond flour

1 tablespoon psyllium husk
½ teaspoon baking powder
Butter to fry in

Mix all of the ingredients except butter, and let sit for a couple of minutes so that the psyllium husk can rise. Fry approximately six small pancakes (they are very filling) in butter in a frying pan on low to medium heat.

Serve with some raspberries and whipped cream, perhaps flavored with vanilla extract.

Three dinners

BROCCOLI MIXED WITH GROUND BEEF AND GORGONZOLA

(approximately 4 servings)

1 onion
1 package of bacon
10 fresh mushrooms
About 1.1 lbs (500 g) ground beef
1 ½ cups (150 g) gorgonzola
1 cup sour cream (34 percent)
Black pepper
Butter to fry in
1 lb (500 g) broccoli
Grated cheese

Fry the onion in butter, add the bacon and mushrooms, and cut into pieces. Then add the ground beef. When it is cooked all the way through, add the gorgonzola and sour cream. Add pepper to taste; you probably won't need salt because the cheese and bacon are very salty.

Place the broccoli in a baking dish. Add the beef mixture and sprinkle with grated cheese. Let it bake in the oven at 350–400 degrees Fahrenheit (175-200 degrees Celsius) for twenty to twenty-five minutes or until the cheese has got a nice color and the broccoli is soft.

Serve with a crispy green salad.

MARIE'S SIMPLE OVEN BAKED FISH (approximately 4 servings)

1 1B (500 G) of frozen mackerel, or alternatively 1.1 lbs (500 g) frozen salmon
Salt and pepper
⅔ cup (400 ml) heavy cream
3-4 tablespoons dill

Defrost the blocks of fish in order to be able to cut them into
slices, about ¾ inch (2 cm) wide. Disperse the fish in a buttered
oven dish; add salt and pepper. Add cream and dill over the fish.
Place in the oven at 350 degrees Fahrenheit (175 degrees Celsius)
for about twenty-five minutes.

Serve with boiled broccoli or another side dish.

McDIET DOCTOR

1 lb (500 g) ground beef
2-3 eggs, depending on size
Salt and pepper
Butter to fry in

Condiments: mayonnaise, lettuce, pickles, fried bacon, onion,
cheese, and oopsie bread (see recipe on p. 205)

Mix the ground beef, eggs, and spices. Form the burgers and fry
them in butter. Build the hamburger on a piece of oopsie bread.
Add a spoonful of mayonnaise, a piece of lettuce, perhaps a slice
of tomato, and a pickle. Add another beef burger and some onion,
bacon, and slices of cheese. Top off with some additional mayonnaise before you place another piece of oopsie on top.

If you want to change things up, you can make the burgers from ground lamb and build it with tzatziki and halloumi
cheese.

CHAPTER ELEVEN

Questions, answers, and myths

Exactly how many carbohydrates should I eat?

The fewer carbohydrates you eat, the more of an effect it will have on your weight, blood sugar, and other things. Try for yourself.

Some tend to feel the best (and become healthier and thinner) from an extremely low amount of carbohydrates, or almost none at all. That is mostly true for middle-aged or older people who are already heavily overweight or who suffer from one of the Western diseases like type 2 diabetes.

Healthy, young, thin people who exercise regularly will be fine with moderate amounts of carbohydrates in their diet. Especially if they eat carbohydrates of good quality and avoid the worst ones: sugar and white flour. Some feel better when they eat fewer carbohydrates. For example, perhaps it calms the stomach or reduces acne.

Some spend a lot of time discussing if 5, 10, 20, or 30 energy percent is the right limit for a low-carbohydrate diet. Such limits are often arbitrary; they have no scientific support. As previously mentioned, sensitivity varies from person to person. If you eat minimal amounts of carbohydrates it becomes extra important *which* carbohydrates you eat. Finally, percentage limits are often useless since most people don't plan their meals according to energy percent nutrition, but based on which food they want. Thus, I am against limits. But I can offer some general guidelines for anyone who wishes.

If you have a difficult time losing weight or suffer from any Western disease, I suggest you eat as few carbohydrates (especially sugar and starch) as you can possibly live with comfortably. For those of you who calculate the nutrition in your diet: 10 energy percent of carbohydrates (about fifty grams per day) has been suggested as the limit for strict LCHF. This can be viewed as an upper limit for those who are carbohydrate-sensitive.

If you want to be really strict, you can stick to under twenty grams of carbohydrates per day. That practically means unlimited amounts of meat, fish, eggs, and butter. Reasonable amounts of above-ground vegetables, cream, and cheese can also fit, but not really any diversions.

With fifty grams of carbohydrates per day, there is room for lots of vegetables, some root vegetables, nuts and berries, more cream, cheese, and some days also a piece of fruit and occasionally a smaller diversion.

Doesn't the brain need at least one hundred grams of carbohydrates per day?

No. That is a funny misconception. Some dietitians and dietary advisors still believe that. That is despite the fact that people have written books (like this one). Those types of things rarely impress these experts. They seem to have their road mapped out and do not want to be interrupted by reality.

Here is the reason behind this misconception: the brain spends about one hundred grams of glucose per day *if* you eat a lot of carbohydrates. If you eat fewer carbohydrates, the brain adjusts to burn mostly fat instead, via ketone bodies. In other words: a significantly increased fat metabolism, even while you are on the couch.

If you eat less than the small amount of glucose that the body is always burning, around twenty grams per day, the liver can produce it from protein in the fat that you consume. You can eat zero grams of carbohydrates a day for as long as you want. Your brain will still work.

Remember the potential withdrawal symptoms though. The first week, before the body has adjusted, some might feel fatigue and unfocused. But it usually passes quickly.

A study randomly selected 106 overweight people to go on either a low-carbohydrate diet (twenty grams per day) or a low-fat diet during an entire year, and measured their wellbeing as well as memory and mental clarity. After a year, those in the low-carbohydrate group felt no different than before, their mental clarity remained unchanged, but their memory had significantly improved throughout the study.

Another study randomly selected ninety-three overweight people to go on either a strict low-carbohydrate diet (around twenty grams per day) or a low-fat diet for eight weeks. The low-carbohydrate group lost the most weight. Those who ate fewer carbohydrates felt happier than before and also scored higher on memory and mental clarity.

These two studies show unchanged or perhaps improved brain functionality on a strict low-carbohydrate diet.

There is one advantage to the misconception that "the brain needs carbohydrates." If someone says that you know that the person has no clue about a low-carbohydrate diet. You can ignore anything else that person says about the subject.

Isn't low-carbohydrate food expensive?
It may be expensive, average, or cheap. If you want to live on filet mignon, lobster tail, and nice wines, it might get expensive. If you buy cheaper meat and fish, it becomes affordable. If you bulk up when there are special offers and freeze it, you will save even more. Eggs are cheap, but it can be worth a couple extra dollars for the organic kind. A lot of butter and cream in your cooking makes you full, so you don't need portions as large as before. Many are surprised by the fact that they can consume much smaller portions and still feel full.

You should also remember the costs that you are avoiding. Ready-made and fast food is expensive, especially if you consider how little nutrition you get for your money. Soda, chocolate, and chips are not free either. You can easily cook a nice low-carbohydrate dinner for your family with good ingredients, for half the price of McDonald's. That doesn't even take into account future healthcare, medications, and dental costs. In addition, it will probably be a lot more fun. If you cook enough food, there should be enough for you to bring to lunch during work. That way you save even more time and money.

Are ketones/ketosis dangerous?

Ketosis is a natural state for humans. As soon as you haven't eaten a lot of carbohydrates in a while, as soon as the insulin runs low, ketones are produced. It is an energy molecule in the blood similar to glucose. Fat is converted into ketones in the liver and become nutrition for the brain. Ketones increase the fat metabolism.

Ketosis is a natural state, since humans used to always risk not having access to food on a regular basis. Go one day without food, and you will be guaranteed to enter ketosis. It might be enough with a good night's worth of sleep; you probably have a few ketones in your blood before breakfast, regardless of what you eat. That is normal. It is not normal to have a fast food restaurant around the corner to always keep the ketones away.

Populations up north, where agriculture was impossible, like Inuits or our Swedish Sami people, always followed a low-carbohydrate diet. They probably went through life in constant ketosis. They were also largely free from our endemic diseases. Ketosis was completely harmless.

Some are still afraid of ketosis. Why? Those who worry about the word ketosis may have confused this natural state with a different, harmful state called ketoacidosis. Ketoacidosis occurs mostly with type 1 diabetics who aren't injecting the insulin they are unable to produce. That results in a *very elevated blood sugar*, but without insulin the body cannot use it. The treatment is rather to inject more insulin.

KETOSIS	KETOACIDOSIS
Normal, healthy	Sickly, dangerous
Among healthy people	Predominantly among type 1 diabetics
Normal blood sugar (approximately 4-7)	**Elevated blood sugar** (above approximately 270 mg/dl)
Normal pH level in the blood	Low pH level in the blood (acidic)
Ketones in the blood	Lots of ketones in the blood
No sugar in the urine	Sugar in the urine
Urine ketones in the blood (sometimes)	Ketones in the urine
Average low insulin	Abnormal insulin deficiency

Ketoacidosis never occurs because of a low-carbohydrate diet. Quite the opposite. A low-carbohydrate diet *reduces the need* for insulin, and ketoacidosis happens when there's an abnormal insulin deficiency.

If someone panics from hearing the word ketosis, you can help. Explain that normal, harmless ketosis is something different from harmful ketoacidosis. Surprisingly, many otherwise knowledgeable people, even doctors, confuse the two.

Do you have to be in ketosis to burn fat?
No. Being in a state of ketosis means you burn fat faster.

How do you know if you are in ketosis?
Especially in the beginning, a few ketones might escape through the lungs and give a characteristic smell to one's breath. It often disappears with time.

Ketones can also escape through the urine and be measured there with a urine stick. Some use this measurement as an indicator that they are eating few enough carbohydrates to remain in a state of ketosis. That is correct, but be mindful that after a time of adjustment, ketones usually don't appear in the urine. You might be in a state of ketosis without the urine stick showing any results.

Do you need to eat carbohydrates to have the energy to work out?
No. But if you are going to compete, you need a reasonable amount in order to win. Carbohydrates are rocket fuel. The problem is that if you eat too much of it, your body becomes wobbly: excess subcutaneous tissue is not an advantage for athletes.

Working out on a low-carbohydrate diet can at best make your muscles really defined, like granite. It can also improve your metabolism, which is good for endurance sports. Prior to and during a competition, you might benefit from increasing your carbohydrate intake. But excess carbohydrate gluttony is hardly necessary even then. Excess pasta consumption days before a competition might make you unnecessarily bloated and heavy at the starting line.

An increasing number of athletes see the advantages of a reasonable low-carbohydrate diet. For example, Björn Ferry who won Olympic gold in biathlon in 2010. The year before, he reduced his carbohydrate consumption from about 60 percent to around 15 percent by giving up pasta, grits, potato, granola, and most types of bread. The result? A body with less subcutaneous fat but more muscles . . . and that gold medal.

Jonas Colting, the star triathlete, has long promoted exercising on a diet consisting of real food without unnecessary sugar and starch. You have to search really hard to find a more chiseled six-pack, and he wins competitions, too.

Recently, Jimmy Lidberg placed in the World Cup in wrestling. In an interview he talked about how he recently had become leaner and more agile, but not lighter. He thanked the new dietary advice he had received: "Fewer carbohydrates and more fat. I have more energy, feel better." As a bonus, his digestive system calmed down.

Ferry, Colting, and Lidberg demonstrate that even elite athletes can exercise without large amounts of carbohydrates. Then it can hardly be an issue for amateurs. Personally, I do weight lifting or go running two or three times a week, and I have noticed the classic effect since I started following a low-carbohydrate diet around five years ago. Less subcutaneous fat and more defined muscles.

Especially if you exercise to achieve weight loss, it is of course a huge benefit to give up sugar and starch. How long does it take? The biggest adjustment takes place during the first couple of weeks, but for some it takes months before the strength and endurance are probably back, especially with a super-strict low-carbohydrate diet.

You have to try for yourself to see which amount of carbohydrates is appropriate to maintain your weight, health, and exercise routine. But do not be surprised if it is less than you thought.

Do you not have to eat a lot of fiber?

Short answer: no. The long answer can be found in the story in chapter two about how Doctor Denis Burkitt launched his fiber theory in the 1970s.

In conclusion, fiber can be good if you are eating large amounts of carbohydrates, since they slow down the absorption thereof. But if you eat fewer carbohydrates, you need fewer fibers. Protein and fat also reduce the uptake of sugar.

Today's excessive belief in fiber is based on many uncertain observational studies. Fiber supplements have no demonstrated health benefit in high-quality studies; the only exception is its ability to ease constipation. The problem with excess fiber intake is that sensitive people might suffer from gas or stomach aches as a result.

In recent years, the junk food industry has finally turned the fiber theory into a farce through its marketing. Of course, heavily sugared breakfast cereal for kids does not become healthier with added fiber and the added words "whole grain" on the box. Even soda has been marketed with a health benefit by containing soluble fiber. That is like putting filters on cigarettes and calling them healthy.

If you want to eat natural fibers to keep your stomach going, I suggest plenty of vegetables instead. Unless it gives you problems with gas.

Do I not have to eat a lot of antioxidants?
No. The theory that antioxidants help against all sorts of diseases is part marketing/advertising and part wishful thinking.

The theory is based on observational studies that do not prove that a correlation is related to a cause. In short: people who eat a lot of vegetables consume more antioxidants than people who subsist on junk food, and the former group is of course much healthier on average. Is it the antioxidants that made them healthy or the thousands of other differences? Of course it is impossible to know.

To be certain, you have to conduct an intervention study. The findings of such studies have not been positive for antioxidants.

A current, extensive review analyzed sixty-seven randomized studies of antioxidant supplements or placebo. It concluded that there was no proven benefit. On the contrary, it showed that an excess of vitamin A, beta carotene, or vitamin E *increases* the risk of premature death!

When the antioxidant theory was eventually tested, everything fell flat. Yet we still talk about the widespread need for them? There are two reasons. One is that it is used as a comfortable word to defend today's low-fat dietary advice. Despite the fact that there are barely any antioxidants in pure sugar or food with a lot of starch.

The second reason is more transparent. Companies want to provide their products with a health aura by using the word antioxidants. They can be added to any type of junk. Is soda with added antioxidants good for you? Of course not, it is a way to trick you into purchasing expensive sugared water.

Through pyramid selling, the message is spread about the almost magical health-improving beverages and the added goji berries, acai, or the fruits noni or mangosteen. The sales representatives throw names of antioxidants around like anthocyanins and polyphenols. Purchasing these expensive products are said to provide a wide array of different health benefits— improving your immune system, protecting against cancer, and detoxing your body—and if you are already healthy you will of course experience more energy, endurance, and "mental clarity." Of course it will also make you thinner, with more youthful skin.

It is just a health bluff. There are no proofs of these miraculous claims about antioxidants. They are the modern "snake oils."

Interestingly enough, our bodies produce our own antioxidants inside our cells (which supplements rarely access) as protection against free radicals. From what I can tell, that seems to suffice. If you still want to make sure you are getting enough antioxidants, you should eat a lot of vegetables. Not junk food with suspect additives, or expensive supplements that may kill you prematurely.

How do you get enough vitamins on a low-carbohydrate diet?
A real low-carbohydrate diet based on meat, fish, eggs, and vegetables is very nutritious, so it is hardly a problem. Many people probably eat more vitamins (and vegetables) than ever before, now that they've started to cook low-carbohydrate food using healthy ingredients.

Eggs are a good example. A growing chicken cannot jump out of the egg shell and have a fruit now and then. All the vitamins needed to build a chicken must be found inside the egg. If you eat an egg, you receive all of them. The Swedish USDA recently analyzed eggs and was surprised by how many vitamins they contain. "There are few other foods that contain such a complete set of vitamins and are so rich in trace materials," said Irene Mattisson, nutritionist, who worked on the study.

Some people say that you need a lot of fruit because of vitamin C. A vitamin C deficiency results in scurvy. But I haven't heard about a scurvy epidemic in recent years, despite the increased popularity of a low-carbohydrate diet. The fact is that the most recent documented Swedish case is said to be from the 1980s.

There are more real dangers than scurvy to worry about. Perhaps the acrylamide in chips or swine flu? If you eat vegetables, for example broccoli or bell peppers, you get plenty of vitamin C.

Is fat or saturated fat (like butter) dangerous?
Short answer: no. See chapter three for the long answer. In conclusion, there is lots of research on the topic suggesting that a reduced intake of fat and saturated fat don't help prevent heart disease.

If you add all the observational studies, people who eat a lot of saturated fat do not suffer from more cardiovascular disease than those who eat a little saturated fat. So the answer is no, the total fat intake or the intake of saturated fat has nothing to do with heart disease.

Is it not important to eat more polyunsaturated fat and less saturated fat?

No. You can put lipstick on a pig, but it is still a pig. Just as the scientific support for the fear of fat is falling apart, the increasingly desperate excuses for still continuing as usual have thrived.

Modern science shows that natural saturated fat is harmless. It has been convincingly documented in new reviews with both observational and intervention studies (see chapter three). Still, some people claim that it is important to "substitute" the harmless saturated fat in one's food. Instead, you are supposed to eat more artificial margarine, made from polyunsaturated fat from plant oils. Something completely new in the human diet.

It is difficult to see the logic in that idea. Of course, some might still want to try to save their credibility when their low-fat diets turn out to be incorrect. Others have big economic interests in today's food industry that are threatened by changing advice. But is there any scientific evidence? Two meta-analyses are usually evoked as support. Plenty of question marks surround them both.

Jacobsen et al (2009) is a strange story. It claims to show that the risk of heart disease is reduced if you "substitute" saturated fat for polyunsaturated fat. But the article analyzes observational studies, not intervention studies! In other words, in reality, no one has been influenced to "substitute" anything. Talking about "substituting" is supported through a complicated statistical crunch of observational data which was already uncertain and couldn't prove causation. With statistical manipulation of numbers, the credibility hardly increases. Even if you trust the numbers, this shows that the same "substitution" of carbohydrates for saturated fat (equal to today's dietary advice) actually *increases* the risk of heart disease. The article is mostly a curiosity in the debate.

Mozzafarian et al. (2010) claim to investigate randomized studies that increase the intake of polyunsaturated fat while simultaneously also decreasing the intake of saturated fat. Collectively, they saw a significantly reduced risk of heart disease. But their choice of studies excluded any of the large studies such as the WHI. The smaller studies that were included were all between eighteen and forty years old. The newest study was published in 1992, which seems odd for a "new" meta-analysis. The only included study that showed a clear positive effect was the so-called Finnish mental hospital study, the design of which was criticized for many reasons. In conclusion, it doesn't fulfill today's scientific requirements. To start, it was not randomized and therefore didn't fulfill the formal criteria to be included in the analysis. Without this non-randomized study conducted in a mental hospital in Finland in the 1960s, there is no correlation.

So it's doubtful science can be a serious foundation for general dietary advice. It is smelling more like desperation. I see no scientific reasons to "substitute" what has proven to be harmless real food for industrially processed plant oil.

Other types of real food with more unsaturated fat such as olives, avocado, and fatty fish are surely good too. But it is not necessarily better. You can eat the real food that you like best with a clear conscience, regardless of how many of the fat molecules are saturated.

What is wrong with margarine?

Margarine is an artificial butter imitation, produced from cheaper ingredients. No health benefits have been documented, despite the commercials. Perhaps the biggest issue with margarine is that it tastes worse than butter. But it could be worse.

Margarine is predominantly produced from cheap plant seed oil, with a very high level of polyunsaturated omega-6. It is worrisome that that type of fat can be transformed into inflammatory compounds inside the body. Small amounts of omega-6 are critical. But during the last couple of decades, the average intake has increased dramatically, along with the industrial production of these cheap and practical fats. Today's intake is probably the highest it has ever been in the Western world.

It is worrisome because we have recently also experienced an epidemic of inflammatory diseases such as asthma, allergies, and eczema. A few intervention studies have pointed to a correlation between a large intake of omega-6-rich margarine and similar diseases. I have listed six of those in the reference section.

Three short examples: A German study showed that many young adults who often ate margarine had a 130 percent increased risk of suffering from asthma. Those who often ate low-fat margarine had a 350 percent increased risk to suffer from asthma. Another study, conducted with two-year-old children, showed that those who used to eat margarine had a 110 percent increased risk of eczema diagnosed by doctors. They also had an increased risk of allergies.

Finally: A new study conducted on over two hundred thousand northern Europeans, including Swedes, showed that those who consumed a lot of omega-6 fat from, for example, margarine, had a 150 percent increased risk of suffering from the inflammatory intestinal disease ulcerous colitis. It can result in disabling stomach aches, intestinal bleeding, and diarrhea. Worst-case scenario, the colon has to be removed.

The studies mentioned above are just observational studies. As per usual, they prove neither causation nor correlation. To know for certain, it takes large, expensive intervention studies. Unfortunately it is unlikely that margarine producers will spend money on finding evidence that their products are dangerous.

Personally, I tend to believe in correlation. I have lost count of how many people describe that their asthma or allergies have improved or disappeared from a natural low-carbohydrate diet (and avoiding margarine). It would be incredibly interesting to see a study on that topic.

There is one additional reason to be skeptical of margarine. It has to do with sincerity. For example, Sweden's largest margarine producer Unilever pretends to not know about the processes that go into producing margarine. In a recent video it posted to You-Tube, they show the ingredients canola oil, palm tree oil, water, lecithin, low-fat sour milk, salt, beta carotene (otherwise the margarine would be white) and lemon juice. They easily whip this all up into margarine, strangely enough in a big bowl of ice water to make the mixture solidify in the video. It all happens "the same way people have always done it in the kitchen" they say.[1]

What they don't tell you is that the included oil gets washed through different processes. Otherwise the margarine would have tasted more like canola or palm tree oil. These processes eradicate any trace of vitamins or similar nutrients. Instead, they add artificial butter flavors.

They also fail to mention that in reality, the oils go through a chemical process called transesterification. This is to transform the liquid oils into fats that can be solid even in room temperature. This process utilizes the extremely reactive sodium ethylate to dissolve the fatty acids and reassemble them in a different way. I emailed Unilever and asked them. They willingly admitted that their table margarine contain transesterified fat.

Do you have sodium ethylate in your kitchen?

What is the difference between GI and LCHF?
GI and LCHF are similar, but LCHF is a tougher diet. The GI diet tells you to reduce your intake of the worst carbohydrates, such as sugar and white flour. LCHF tells you to significantly reduce your intake of all carbohydrates.

The GI diet advocates for the consumption of complex carbohydrates such as whole grain pasta products. On the LCHF diet you eat predominantly meat, fish, eggs, butter, and vegetables.

The advantage of GI is that it is more forgiving if you like bread and pasta, and you avoid withdrawal symptoms such as fatigue and headaches the first couple of days.

The advantage with LCHF is that it causes more effective weight loss, more stable blood sugar, and decreased cravings for sugar.

---

1. You can equate this production with real butter. Then you simply just whisk cream long enough until it becomes butter. No suspect bowl of ice water is needed to make such a video.

Is it enough to eat carbohydrates with a low GI?
For healthy, thin, young, and physically strong people: yes, perhaps. For overweight people and diabetics: probably not. At least it is much less effective.

Pay attention to things that have the words "whole grain" on the package, such as different kinds of bread or pasta, since they are often just partially made from whole grains. The rest is white flour, as per usual.

Also don't miss the biggest flaw with GI: sugar (sucrose) has a pretty low GI, since sugar is half fructose that slowly raises the blood sugar. But fructose in larger amounts seems to be the "best" there is to gain weight and suffer from metabolic syndrome. Watch out for food with lots of sugar/fructose, even if the glycemic index is okay.

Can carbohydrates in food turn into fat in the body?
Sure, especially fructose, which is easily transformed into fat in the liver. An excess of carbohydrates that spikes the insulin also risks resulting in an increased storage of the fat that you are consuming.

Do I really need to eat fatty food? Is it not enough to eat more fruit, greens, and fiber?
No, it is not enough. If you want to significantly reduce the sugar and starch, you need energy from something else in order to be satisfied.

Above-ground vegetables or fiber contain very little energy. You don't get long-term satisfaction from them. Your stomach might feel full, but that is not the same thing. You will soon feel hungry again. Fruit is somewhat richer in energy, but it is in forms of sugar. That is why it is best to eat the fruit you want, because it is tasty. Fruit is natural candy.

To feel full without sugar and starch, you need fat, the most energy-rich nutrition there is. Of course that doesn't mean you have to "stuff yourself with fat." Fat is very filling, so no large portions are required. You have to let go of your fear of fat.

How much fat is reasonable? Enough to feel full.

What is the difference between a low-carbohydrate diet and the paleo diet?
The difference between the paleo diet and today's low-carbohydrate diet is that the former also excludes dairy products. During the Stone Age, we didn't keep animals and didn't drink milk after we were weaned. We didn't have cream, cheese, or butter.

The main reason for accepting dairy products in a low-carbohydrate diet today is that it makes life simpler and tastier. Sugar and starch are the new problem that has to be avoided. Fatty dairy products seem harmless. But if you are satisfied without dairy products, a strict paleo diet is an excellent choice.

How can Japanese people be so thin when they eat so much rice?
A common question. A couple of populations have traditionally consumed high levels of carbohydrates without suffering from obesity. They share three traits.

First of all, they barely eat any pure sugar. A lot of fructose from sugar can catalyze the process that produces constantly high insulin levels. Secondly, they eat unrefined starch with a low GI. Finally, these populations were generally poor, lacked an excess of food, and engaged in heavy physical labor.

During these three conditions, most people seem to tolerate a high portion of indigestible starch in their diets without becoming obese. When it comes to Japanese people, it is also noteworthy that a common saying is *hara hachi bu* or "eat until you are 80 percent full." Perhaps there is risk of overeating brown rice as well?

Even if many people can remain thin on a raw starch-rich diet (without sugar), the developments usually don't turn around for those who are already obese or have type 2 diabetes. They might require a strict low-carbohydrate diet.

Finally, it is interesting to see what Japanese Sumo wrestlers traditionally eat. They have consistently tried to refine their diets to become heavy. They eat very little fat. According to a study published in *American Journal of Clinical Nutrition*, young Sumo wrestlers eat on average 1003 grams of carbohydrates per day, but only fifty grams of fat.

Should I follow a low-carbohydrate diet if I am of average weight?

Yes. People of average weight may notice reduced subcutaneous fat, but only lose as much as the body thinks is enough. Conversely, underweight people might add more muscle weight.

You don't have to eat bread or sugar to maintain a normal weight. It is enough to eat until you are full. An unlimited low-carbohydrate diet is not a regular weight loss diet. If you are overweight you will shed pounds, but if you are underweight you will gain some. A low-carbohydrate diet is a long-term method for weight control.

Can I follow a low-carbohydrate diet if I am pregnant or breast-feeding?

There are no medical reasons why you should eat the new food, sugar and pure starch, at any point in your life.

A natural and varied low-carbohydrate diet with meat, fish, butter, eggs, and plenty of vegetables, along with nuts and berries, is very nutritious. It should be excellent food even when you are eating for two. I recommend eating varied types of food and plenty of it. Positive effects on the mother, such as on her weight, should be seen as a side effect during pregnancy and breastfeeding. The most important thing is, of course, that the baby is healthy—but it ought to be a good sign if the mother is as well.

When it comes to a strict low-carbohydrate diet, there are no studies that have examined the effect during pregnancy or breastfeeding. According to a new review of the scientific evidence, there is also published data that demonstrates the minimal requirement of carbohydrates for pregnant women.

Everything comes down to the fact that science doesn't have the answer when it comes to a strict low-carbohydrate diet. You have to judge the risk for yourself by eating different things during a pregnancy or while breast feeding.

An excess amount of blood sugar-raising carbohydrates could obviously be detrimental for someone who is overweight or suffers from high blood pressure. Many pregnant women put on too much weight. Gestational diabetes is also common today, and that often results in an abnormally large baby. That demonstrates the risk with the conventional Western diet.

A strict low-carbohydrate diet might also be dangerous in other ways, even if those effects remain unknown. Anecdotally, it seems to be fine and no cases of side effects have been published. But science doesn't have the final answer. Therefore it may be wise to consume at least some carbohydrates through vegetables, berries, nuts, and dairy products.

Can I eat carbohydrates if I am also taking medicine X?
LEVOTHYROXINE: Yes. But some might need to adjust their dosage in the long run (often reduce it, sometimes, increase it).

WARFARIN: Regardless of any dietary change you make while on Warfarin, you should contact whoever conducts your Warfarin tests in order to get tested more frequently. You might need to adjust your dosage.

BLOOD PRESSURE MEDICATION: Yes, but be prepared that your blood pressure might be reduced from a low-carbohydrate diet. Then you might need to contact your doctor to adjust (decrease) the dosage. Regular symptoms are dizziness or fatigue.

DIABETES MEDICATION: A low-carbohydrate diet is excellent for diabetics. But you have to be careful with your medication in order to keep your blood sugar from plummeting (metformin is the only medication that does not increase the risk of hypoglycemia). Usually the dosage must be reduced. Many diabetics need to reduce their insulin doses by 30 percent or more when they avoid carbohydrates. The dietary change should take place in agreement with your doctor or diabetes nurse.

Can I follow a low-carbohydrate diet when I have reduced kidney functionality?

If you have significantly reduced kidney functionality (on the verge of requiring dialysis), you may have received the advice to avoid protein. Then you should keep doing that. Otherwise, there is to my knowledge nothing that should keep you from following a low-carbohydrate diet.

A randomized study with sixty-eight obese participants has examined this particular scenario. After a couple of years on a low-carbohydrate diet or high-carbohydrate diet, there was no difference between the two groups' kidney functionality. The trend was toward *improved* kidney functionality in the low-carbohydrate group throughout the study.

A dramatic patient case was published in Swedish medical news a couple of years ago. A sixty-year-old man with type 2 diabetes had long suffered from renal failure. He began insulin treatment in 1997 and he gained more and more weight, while his kidney functionality declined. In January of 2004 he started following a low-carbohydrate diet. His blood sugar improved radically, and he was able to go off the insulin injections within a couple of weeks. He shed 42 lbs (19 kg) the first six months, then a couple of additional ones. His kidney functionality, which had been declining, stabilized. His kidney functionality was seemingly better at his three-year checkup.

Diabetes is the most common reason behind renal failure in Sweden today. There is no doubt that a low-carbohydrate diet has an excellent effect on elevated blood sugar.

Can I follow a low-carbohydrate diet if I suffer from gallbladder issues?

That is usually fine. Fatty food might cause gallbladder attacks if you already suffer from gallstones. But gallstones are usually a result of low-fat food. Let me explain.

Bile is predominantly produced to dissolve fatty food. If you eat a lot of fatty food, you produce a lot of bile, which flows freely through the bile ducts. This prevents the creation of gallstones.

If you follow a low-fat diet, you produce very little bile. Then the bile risks getting stuck in the bile ducts for long periods of time. This increases the risk of forming stones.

Gallstones are similar to kidney stones. If you have a tendency to suffer from kidney stones, you are advised to drink a lot of water so that you produce urine that rinses out the urinary tract. If you drink too little, the urine is left in the urinary tract and might form kidney stones.

Gallstones work in a similar way. If drinking a lot of water works to help prevent kidney stones, fatty food will protect in the same way against the formation of gallstones.

If you already suffer from gallstones, an increased production of bile from fatty food might cause temporary discomfort. The stones that have already formed might hurt on their way out.

Regularly eating fatty food produces a liberal production of bile, which "flushes out" the bile ducts. If you are lucky, small stones are transported into the intestines and disappear. Those who have followed a LCHF diet a long time seem to be free from gallbladder issues. People who experience temporary discomfort at first can try eating less fat in each meal, but more often, until the stomach hopefully adjusts.

If you have already removed your gallbladder, the bile is directly transported from the bile ducts to the intestines when needed. The ready-made bile is no longer stored in the gallbladder to be used when needed.

In theory, this should mean you have a more difficult time digesting large amounts of fat at a time. In practice, it seems to work just as well, at least when your body has had some time to adjust.

Might I feel unwell at first?

Yes. That is a result of what is called adjustment or withdrawal issues in the form of headaches, fatigue, dizziness, heat flashes, heart palpitations, bad breath, and irritation. It usually passes relatively quickly. A possible effect on your breath, most often in the beginning, is a result of ketosis (see p. 214).

Can I feel more intoxicated from alcohol when I follow a low-carbohydrate diet?
Yes. Many people who follow a low-carbohydrate diet experience an elevated sense of intoxication from alcohol. Be careful if you don't know your limit.

The cause is unknown. Perhaps it is because alcohol is dissolved in the liver, similar to fructose (that is the reason why excess amounts of alcohol and fructose can result in fatty liver). With a low-carbohydrate diet, you eat very little fructose and the liver might, as a result, be unaccustomed to dissolving it. Another alternative is that the liver is busy producing blood sugar and ketones and therefore dissolves the alcohol more slowly.

Might I experience leg cramps from a low-carbohydrate diet?
Yes. Some have issues with leg cramps in the beginning of following a low-carbohydrate diet. The reason could be the loss of magnesium in the kidney in conjunction with the change. That seems to adjust itself with time.

If you have issues, it seems to help to ingest magnesium supplement for a while, approximately 400 milligrams per day.

Might I feel constipated from following a low-carbohydrate diet?
Yes. Some people experience constipation in the beginning. Some also experience the opposite, diarrhea. The stomach needs time to adjust to a large dietary change.

The most important thing to prevent constipation is to drink enough water. If you become dehydrated, your body absorbs more fluids from the large intestine, which produces harder feces and risk of constipation.

A reduced intake of fiber could also result in constipation before the stomach adjusts. You can prevent this by eating lots of fiber-rich vegetables.

Will I suffer from osteoporosis from following a low-carbohydrate diet?

No. The reason for this concern is that some studies have showed reduced bone density among children whose epilepsy has been treated with a low-carbohydrate diet, *compared to healthy children*. But those kids have also been treated with high doses of various epilepsy medications. Some medications list osteoporosis as a side effect. Thus, the children risk osteoporosis regardless of diet. A vitamin D deficiency might also contribute.

There are no signs that our ancestors or populations that traditionally followed a low-carbohydrate diet suffered from osteoporosis; in fact, quite the opposite is evident.

A couple of studies have examined the effect of low-carbohydrate diets on the bones. In the first study, fifteen people were asked to follow a strict low-carbohydrate diet for three months. Compared to the control group, there were no signs of a disrupted bone turnover in specific urine and blood tests.

In the second study, 307 obese participants were randomly selected to follow either a low-carbohydrate or low-fat diet for almost two years. They compared the two groups at six, twelve, and twenty-four months in terms of bone density in their vertebral columns and hips, among other things. Neither of the groups displayed any change in bone density throughout the study.

A low-carbohydrate diet doesn't cause osteoporosis.

Can I get colon cancer from red meat?

Most likely, no. The fear of a correlation between cancer and eating fat or meat has not been supported by modern studies. The by far largest intervention study WHI showed no decreased risk of cancer when half of fifty thousand women were randomly selected to follow a low-fat diet with more fruit and vegetables.

The only concern that remains is whether or not red meat can cause colon cancer. That is based on correlations in observational studies, which do not show causation. It has been discussed whether these statistical correlations have to do with the added preservative nitrite in meat products.

In a recent review of these observational studies, the correlations between red meat and colon cancer are pretty weak. They become even less credible by the fact that meat-eaters statistically eat more sugar and smoke more, etc. Other lifestyle factors may therefore be behind the statistical correlations. In conclusion, they saw no evidence of correlation between red meat and colon cancer when they added all of the studies.

On the other hand, many observational studies have showed clearer correlations between carbohydrate intake, a heavy glycemic strain, and various forms of cancer. See the section about cancer in the chapter about Western diseases.

Do you have more questions?
More questions and answers can be found at www.Dietdoctor.com.

CHAPTER TWELVE

How to lose weight

M any people who follow a low-carbohydrate diet do so in order to lose weight. Often, it works perfectly from the start. But some wish it happened faster, or they get stuck after some time with a stagnated weight loss and want to lose more.

How do you improve your weight loss? Here are seventeen of my best pieces of advice. The most important advice is listed in the beginning, so the farther you get down the list, the less important or rare the problems are. So please pay extra attention to the advice listed at the top.

1. Choose a low-carbohydrate diet

Forget a calorie-limiting low-fat diet. After having read this book, you know how poorly it performs in the long run and how easily you end up yo-yo dieting if you cannot ever feel full. A large number of studies have demonstrated that you lose more weight from following a low-carbohydrate diet, without even having to count calories or being hungry.

A common pace is a couple of pounds the first week, and thereafter about one pound per week. About 55 lbs (25 kg) per year is a normal result, if you completely give up sugar or starch. The stricter you are, the better the effect usually is. When you approach your body's ideal weight, the weight loss slows down, in order to stabilize at a level where the body feels comfortable. You will never become underweight if you eat until you are satisfied.

Of course, the pace varies from individual to individual. Younger men tend to lose weight more quickly. Older women usually lose weight more slowly. Unfortunately, the world is unfair.

2. Be patient

For many people, it took years or decades to put on the extra pounds. It is usually significantly quicker to get rid of them. But you need to be patient.

Eat well, feel good, and distract yourself with something else. Feel free to get rid of your scale. A low-carbohydrate diet is not a quick starvation diet. It is a long-term lifestyle. The hormonal environment in your body changes when the insulin level decreases. With time, your body is reshaped; the abdominal fat slowly disappears. Sooner or later, another pair of pants will fit loosely.

There are plenty of miracle promises in magazines and online, for about $70 plus shipping. That only decreases the size of your wallet. Spend your money on real food instead and give it some time. If you lose pounds every month, you will eventually become thin. That is inevitable. A pound a week might sound like just a little, but that is 55 lbs (25 kg) per year.

Be prepared to sometimes drop a couple of pounds every couple of days, while sometimes your weight is at a standstill for a week. Temporary stagnations on the way down are so common I don't think I have ever met someone who hasn't experienced them.

You need patience. But please continue reading. There are things you can do to maximize your weight loss.

3. Eat enough fat

What is the most common mistake for a beginner following a low-carbohydrate diet? Simple. They are still afraid of fat.

Fewer carbohydrates without more fat results in starvation. You will become hungry and tired. In the end, you are ready to give up. Please avoid this pitfall. In order to become thin in the long run, you must be comfortable and feel good about your food.

The solution is simple: eat yourself full with fat. Fry your food in butter and add liberal amounts of cream to your sauces. Fatty meat, fish, bacon, eggs, coconut fat, and avocado are great sources for feeling full.

If you are still hungry, you have eaten too little fat. Always eat enough to feel satisfied, especially in the beginning. With time, naturally fatty food will feel like the most normal thing in the world. But in the beginning, many people need to get used to it. As long as you don't trick your body's ability to regulate your appetite with sugar or starch, you will only want to eat just enough. With sufficiently low levels of insulin, it is almost impossible to increase your fat weight. If you eat more now, you will feel satisfied longer, or eat less during the next meal.

Don't be afraid of fat. Natural fat is your friend. You might have another enemy in the beginning: the scale.

4. Focus on your waist measurement

Conventional calorie-counting, quasi starvation, could cause loss of lean muscle mass and might even have an effect on the size of your organs. If you start eating enough to feel full again, that is quickly restored. You often gain weight again.

Even if you start transferring to a low-carbohydrate diet after that, our deficiencies might be restored and your weight might increase in the beginning. But increased body fat can be minimized with a low-carbohydrate diet. Restoring your muscle mass is also good, both for your health and appearance.

The point is that your weight is an arbitrary measurement, especially if you have just been on a starvation diet. There is a better way of measuring your progress.

Your waist measurement, measured with a measuring tape, says more. Always measure the same area in order to be able to compare. I suggest you measure at a level between your hip bone and low rib. Exhale and relax; do not suck in your stomach. Those who are particularly curious can also measure other areas, around your buttocks, chest, arms, and legs. Write down the values so that you can compare a couple of times a month. Between those comparisons it might be enough to feel your pants fit more loosely.

You should utilize the scale less often. For many people, their weight decreases quickly when following a low-carbohydrate diet. But for others—especially those who previously counted calories—the scale might be tricking you. This is caused by the body's attempt to reshape itself due to how the diet is affecting one's hormone levels, especially the insulin.

Do you want a quickly reduced waist measurement? There are a couple of things to note.

5. Women: avoid eating fruit

This goes for men as well, but it is a common obstacle for women who are trying to lose weight.

Unfortunately, fruit contains a lot of sugar, about 10 percent of the weight (the rest is mostly water). Five fruits per day, as many people eat, equals as much as half a liter of soda. It is the same type of sugar.

The sugar contained in the fruit elevates your blood insulin, which might turn off your fat metabolism. Worst-case scenarios, it causes weight gain. Fruit contains relatively low amounts of calories, but the fructose might make you crave other things.

You achieve better results without fruit. If you suffer from weight issues, you should only eat fruit occasionally because it is tasty.

6. Men: avoid drinking beer

This also goes for women, but is a more common obstacle for men. Beer contains a lot of malt sugar, which turns off the fat metabolism. There are good reasons why it is called beer belly.

Better choices of alcohol if you want to lose weight:
• Dry wines (regular red wine, dry white wines)
• Dry champagne
• Hard liquor such as scotch, cognac, vodka (avoid sweet drinks)

They contain a lot less sugar. But even alcohol itself seems to affect weight. It is metabolized in the liver, similar to fructose. Sticking to normal consumption is probably best. Or refrain from it, if you really want to maximize your weight loss.

7. See through the fake products

How about low-carb pasta? Low-carb ice cream? Low-carb chips? Low-carb chocolate?

Can you eat special versions of the carbohydrate-rich junk food without affecting your weight? Unfortunately, no. If it sounds too good to be true, it usually is. These products usually contain plenty of carbohydrates when you scrutinize them. Some are also filled with sugar alcohols and sweeteners. See the section "The snake in paradise" in the initial guidance chapter.

You become healthy and thin from real food, remember that.

8. Avoid sweeteners

Many people replace sugar with sweeteners and believe that the reduced number of calories will enable them to lose weight Perhaps it works sometimes. But studies have shown that people who consume diet soda seem to become just as fat as those who drink regular sugared soda. Several studies conducted on rats have even shown *increased* weight gain from drinking sweeteners instead of sugar.

Some people believe the cause is that the body increases the insulin production when it expects sugar to appear in the blood. When it doesn't, the blood sugar plummets and you feel hungrier. Alternatively, sweeteners stimulate one's craving for sweets and results in snacking.

Regardless, if you have a difficult time losing weight, I suggest you avoid sweeteners. Then you wean off your desire for everything tasting sweet. Your sweet tooth will then disappear in a matter of days.

9. Review your medications

Many medications affect your weight. Of course you should discuss any potential changes with your doctor.

INSULIN INJECTIONS are the worst thing for your weight, especially in large doses. Your insulin requirement might be minimized with a low-carbohydrate diet, which enables weight loss. Metformin pills are usually a good idea for type 2 diabetes. They don't cause weight gain, and might reduce the need for weight-gaining insulin.

OTHER DIABETES MEDICATIONS, such as insulin-raising pills (so called sulfonylurea medications) often cause weight gain. Pills such as Actos, Starlix, and Prandin also cause weight gain. The new medicine Byetta (injection form) actually generates weight loss.

CORTISONE IN PILL FORMAT, such as Prednisone, causes long-term weight gain, especially in high dosages. The dosage should be carefully adjusted to the lowest level that is still effective. Local treatment with cortisone cream, nose spray, or inhalation hardly affects the weight.

Aside from the three worst medications, the following medications might also interrupt your weight loss:

NEUROLEPTICA antipsychotics often causes weight gain. Newer medicines are often worse. Zyprexa (olanzapine) is notorious for causing severe weight gain.

CERTAIN ANTI-DEPRESSANTS, especially older tricyclical medications (e.g. amitriptyline, nortriptyline, clomipramine) as well as Remeron (mirtazapine) and Lithium often cause weight gain. The most common antidepressants, so-called selective serotonin reuptake inhibitors (e.g. citalopram, sertraline), barely affect weight at all.

CERTAIN BIRTH CONTROL medications can cause slight weight gain, especially those that only contain progesterone and not estrogen. Some examples include mini pills, contraceptive injections, or contraceptive rod implants.

BLOOD PRESSURE MEDICATION in forms of beta-blockers can cause weight gain. Some examples are metoprolol and atenolol.

EPILEPSY MEDICATION can cause weight gain, such as Tegretol (carbamazepine) and Depakote (valproate).

ALLERGY MEDICATIONS SUCH as antihistamines can cause weight gain, especially in high doses.

There are also weight-loss medications. At the time this book was written, there was only one such prescription drug in Sweden:

XENICAL (also called Alli in a weaker, prescription-free format)
I discourage the use of Xenical and Alli. They block the uptake of fat in the intestine. They cause diarrhea if you eat real food and also have a limited effect on your weight. A low-carbohydrate diet produced better results in a randomized study alone than fat and calorie restrictions with Xenical.

The future of dieting medication could be so-called GLP 1 ag-onists. They are already prescribed to type 2 diabetics, with the name Byetta or Victoza. They are still relatively untested.

10. Don't stress too much, and get enough sleep

Stress and a poor sleep cycle can affect the levels of the hormone cortisol and cause weight gain. If you have a difficult time losing weight, you are wise to reduce stress and get enough sleep.

If you snore or suffer from sleep apnea (pauses in breathing during sleep), a CPAP machine might help you lose weight more easily—since it produces better sleep and fewer stress hormones. When you eventually lose weight, the snoring usually stops.

11. Feel free to exercise

Exercising is good for your health and wellbeing. It is usually only a bonus for your weight. See the section about exercise in chapter five.

If you suffer from obesity or aches, I suggest you wait to exer-cise. Don't wear out your joints. As you lose more weight, your en-ergy usually returns. When you feel you have some leftover energy, when a walk seems appealing, then you should start.

When you eat until you are full, you get more energy. When your energy storage isn't trapped by high insulin levels, you shouldn't be surprised if you *want* to move more. Do the kinds of things you enjoy and make you feel good. Build up your strength and improve your posture and overall shape. Better health and wellbeing usually comes as a bonus. With time, it might make your body more tolerant of carbohydrates, without raising insulin levels. That might have an improved effect on your weight in the long run—a positive feedback cycle.

12. Eat just enough

Can you really eat *unlimited* amounts of low-carbohydrate food and still lose weight? Yes, for most people that works well. That means their appetite works and they automatically eat just enough by following their feelings of hunger and satisfaction.

But for some people, it might not be quite that easy. It is actually rare to be able to increase one's body fat above the average level when you are following a low-carbohydrate diet. But with too large of a food intake, their body has no reason to let go of its body fat either. It burns the fat you consume instead of what is in your abdomen. That generates slow weight loss.

If your weight stagnates for a long period of time and you cannot find another solution, this might be the culprit. You can be eating more than you need in order to feel full because it is pleasant and tasty. Common culprits:

Dairy products
Cream
Cheese
Nuts

Please note that none of these (not even nuts in large amounts) used to be common paleo food. They also contain a small amount of carbohydrates. Dairy, milk, and yogurt contain a surprisingly high amount of lactose. Lactose doesn't taste very sweet and can easily be overlooked. Some also think that dairy products can affect weight via milk protein that releases extra insulin. That is a possibility.

If necessary, you can avoid these types of food to see if it helps your weight loss. Then you can try one at a time to see if you tolerate them without obstructing your weight loss.

13. Ensure you have minimized the amount of carbohydrate

If you have a hard time losing weight, you can aim to consume a maximum of twenty grams' worth of carbohydrates per day. These should predominantly derive from vegetables.

Some people may do better with an extremely low amount of carbohydrates, as close to zero as it gets for a certain period. Then you almost exclusively eat meat, fish, eggs, and butter. It is of course crucial to find a way to eat that makes you feel comfortable in the long run. For most people, a zero-carbohydrate period only works temporarily.

14. Consider your hormones

Some people, especially women, may experience a sluggish metabolism as a result of a shortage of their thyroid hormones. Common symptoms are fatigue, feelings of coldness, constipation, and dry skin. That might cause a couple of pounds of weight gain. A blood test at the closest clinic can make that diagnosis. The treatment is often thyroid hormone replacement tablets.

Other sex hormones that affect weight:

• During menopause, the estrogen levels decrease in women, which might cause weight gain.
• Even men experience decreased levels of the sex hormone, testosterone, with age. That can lead to abdominal weight gain (viciously called an old man belly).

Post-middle age, it is almost impossible to become as thin as you were during your teenage years. Changing hormone levels could be the main reason that many older people, especially women, have a difficult time maintaining their weight. When there is an evident deficiency, additional sex hormones are sometimes prescribed. Such supplements could unfortunately have negative long-term health risks, at least in high doses. There are similarities with doping.

15. Take plenty of vitamins and minerals

This lacks research even more. But it is possible that foods with poor sources of nutrition, with a vitamin and mineral deficiency, risk causing overeating. That is a reasonable thought. If you eat food with poor nutrition contents, the body might need to increase its food intake to still get what it requires.

The most exciting study was published in 2010. Around a hundred Chinese women were randomly divided into three groups. For the first six months, the first group received multivitamin supplements, the second group only received calcium, and the third group received a placebo. None of them knew what they were getting, not even their doctors.

After six months, the group that received multivitamins had lost the most weight (on average about 6.3 lbs [3 kg] more) and had the most improved health markers. The calcium supplement had no apparent effect.

It is probably enough to eat nutritious food. But if you experience weight issues, it doesn't hurt to ingest a reasonable dose of daily multivitamins. You can see it as bootstraps.

One specific vitamin is normally too low in multivitamin pills: vitamin D. Vitamin D deficiency is common in Sweden and even more so among obese people. A randomized study of women with vitamin D deficiency and reduced insulin sensitivity showed improved insulin sensitivity from supplements compared to a placebo. That might mean that a vitamin D supplement improves weight loss among some people.

Avoiding vitamin D deficiency has several other health benefits. The increased number of studies on this area is the subject of the next chapter.

16. Eat slower, enjoy more

Some studies indicate that people who eat too quickly consume too much food before they know they are full. Some studies have also shown that overweight people often eat more quickly than thin people. Those are observational studies and do not prove causation, so approach those findings with caution. Junk food is of course bad for several other reasons: it contains lots of sugar and starch.

But if you have weight issues and eat quickly, try to eat slower, and make sure you notice when you are full. Take the time to fully enjoy your food.

17. Try intermittent fasting

Of course you don't have to eat immediately when you feel hungry. The body is designed to handle short periods without food perfectly well. It used to be more common to have periods with less food. Letting the body fast (and only drink water) from time to time could possibly have positive effects on your weight. It hardly hurts to try.

There are different versions of intermittent fasting. Some eat once a day, preferably at night. One more extreme form is to only eat every other day. To my knowledge, neither of these methods have been scientifically tested.

If you are curious, I suggest that you experiment. Skip lunch or breakfast from time to time if it feels okay. If you follow a low-carbohydrate diet, the resulting longer-lasting feeling of satisfaction usually makes it feel okay. It will probably speed up the weight loss. Perhaps it is also healthy.

In conclusion

If you have made it this far, please read advice numbers two and four again.

If you have questions about weight loss or want to discuss with others, I recommend the discussion forum at Dietdoctor.com.

CHAPTER THIRTEEN

One last thing

T he food revolution might produce a new type of health. But there is one more thing that is required in order to maximize it. One more thing that the body needs that is difficult to get from food. One more thing of which we have recently become unnaturally afraid.

Sun

We in Sweden live in the dark Nordics, where the sun only rises high in the sky for a couple of months throughout the year. Aside from that, we are also most often indoors working. Or we avoid going outside with bare skin out of fear of cancer. Many people put on clothes or put on sunscreen to block the few rays of real sun they get all year long.

That is extremely unnatural. Is there a health risk from acting like a cave-residing, light-sensitive Gollum? Yes, recent research has shown an evident risk. It is called vitamin D deficiency, and it is incredibly common in Sweden today.

Your skin produces lots of vitamin D when it is reached by sunlight. You also get a tad bit of it from your diet, especially from fatty fish, but in much smaller doses. Those who avoid the sun experience severe vitamin D deficiency.

Why are native Swedes pale, while people from more southern countries have darker skin? The answer is undoubtedly vitamin D. Darker pigment is a type of built-in sunscreen. We needed to develop paler and lighter sensitive skin in order to live healthily in the dark northern European countries. That is, in order to get the vitamin D that our health requires. If the sun was dangerous, Swedes would have been dark-skinned, like our ancestors that emigrated from Africa.

If we ignore that for which our bodies are designed, we risk disease. That doesn't only mean with regards to food, but also the sun.

What is vitamin D?

Vitamin D is a unique vitamin. It is also a steroid hormone, like our sex hormones testosterone and estrogen, and affects the functionality of hundreds of genes in most of the body's cells. Vitamin D could therefore potentially have any kind of effect on the body.

The common vitamin D deficiency can theoretically increase the risk of several different diseases. An increasing volume of research tends to support this theory. Infectious diseases such as cold and the flu, cancer, heart disease, osteoporosis, autism, general aches/fibromyalgia, winter and spring depression can increase—the list of correlated diseases is long.

In Sweden we easily replenish the vitamin D repository in the summer sun. But then the level in the body slowly decreases. If we don't go on a sunny vacation, we often experience vitamin D deficiency come the winter or spring.

A lot of things still remain to be proven, but it is as good as clear right now. It is wise to have a normal amount of vitamin D in your blood, a level that looks like people who experience intense sunlight from time to time. That might prevent several diseases and there are no known risks for healthy people.

The evidence

We have long known that people with vitamin D deficiency have an increased risk of several diseases. Lots of observational studies have proven this. But they don't show causation. The correlation could just as easily stem from the fact that sick people aren't exposed to sunlight to the same extent. These studies don't show what is the chicken and what is the egg.

To know for sure, you have to conduct randomized intervention studies. Studies that give one group vitamin D supplements and one group a placebo. An increasing number of these studies are being conducted today, and the findings are astonishing.

The most exciting result is that a vitamin D supplement might prolong life. When they compared the accumulated results of eighteen studies where they had prescribed either vitamin D or a placebo, those who had received the supplement lived longer, and that was a statistically significant difference.

Another study conducted on elderly people in the northern United States showed a significantly reduced risk of cancer among the group that received the supplement. Similar studies have indicated a positive effect on depression, the flu, and prevention of osteoporosis.

If we leave the high-quality studies behind, there are a couple that indicate that athletes perform better without a vitamin D deficiency in the blood. Interestingly, doctors for the American ice hockey team Chicago Blackhawks recently began testing and treating vitamin D deficiency in the players. The following year, the players won the Stanley Cup for the first time in forty-nine years. My guess is that the players kept taking vitamin D supplements after that.

But there is one significantly more important reason to avoid a deficiency, or risk a lifelong handicap: autism, in a less severe state called Asperger's syndrome. It is a disturbance in the brain development that, among other things, results in reduced social skills.

In the last couple of decades, this disturbance has become increasingly more common in Sweden and the rest of the Western world. The reason for this is unknown, but several observational studies show that vitamin D deficiency among pregnant women or small children correlates with the development of autism.

The people who suffer the highest risk of vitamin D deficiency in the dark Nordic countries are dark-skinned people and people who because of covering clothes aren't exposed to a lot of sunlight. One example is immigrant Muslim women from Somalia. Their children often suffer from autism. Swedish-Somalian people call this "the Swedish disease."

A couple of years ago, two chief physicians wrote an op-ed in *DN Debatt* in which they discussed the health risks of vitamin D deficiency and suggested an extensive informational campaign to the part of the population that risks the most severe deficiency. Supplements are cheap and harmless, they claimed, and ended with, "So what are we waiting for?"

Nothing has happened since then.

Two glasses of sunlight

So vitamin D is produced when the sun shines on us. But in Sweden the sun is only strong enough during the summer months. The sun must rise above a forty-five-degree angle in order for the right wavelengths to avoid being filtered away in the atmosphere. That means your shadow has to be shorter than you in order for your body to produce vitamin D.

During fifteen minutes in strong sunlight, the body produces more vitamin D than you need over a couple of days. Thus, you don't have to lie down and get burned—not at all. It is enough with reasonable and healthy sun habits. Sunscreen risks providing a false sense of security and tricks us into staying in the sun too long, by stopping rays of sunlight that make the skin red and by letting through others. Perhaps it is better to tan carefully without sunscreen.

We may have been overly warned about the sun, but also shouldn't tan in excess. Ola Larkö, professor of dermatology, compares tanning to drinking wine. Both are positive for your health in small doses. "But tan two glasses a day, not a bottle," he says.

Cure the deficiency

In Sweden, it is wise to take vitamin D supplements during the winter. At least if you don't eat a lot of fatty fish (¾ lbs [350 g] per day or more) or go on a vacation in the sun. It might be extra important for people with darker skin, or people who don't like being out in the sun in the summer.

Vitamin D is cheap, safe, and has no side effects in higher doses. Old recommendations are obsolete today. Unfortunately, there are no supplements with proper doses for adults in the pharmacy. Vitamin D supplements are very cheap and cannot be patented. It is therefore difficult for the industry to make big profits, so there is also no money for advertising.

But you can easily access vitamin D supplements in health stores or online. The following doses will cost you about twenty to thirty cents per day for an adult. To avoid deficiency during the winter:

- Adults: 2000–4000 IU per day
- Children under ten years: 1000 IU daily

If you are a large man, 4,000 calories might be enough, and if you are a small woman, 2,000 calories might be enough. That equates to a couple of minutes in strong sunlight. For healthy people, these doses provide no risk of potentially overdosing.[2]

Some intense sunlight during the summer, possible supple-

---

2. For people with a couple of rare diseases, the normalized vitamin D level might increase the calcium levels in the blood. If you suffer from any of these diseases and increase your tanning or vitamin D supplements, you should ask your doctor to check your calcium levels:

- Hormone-producing tumor in the parathyroid gland
- Granulomatosis diseases such as sarcoidosis or tuberculosis
- Certain types of cancer such as lung cancer and non-Hodgkins lymphoma

ments during the winter, and fatty fish throughout the year. That is the best way of maintaining the proper amount of sun hormone in your body and maximizing your chances of good health.

See you

Eat real food and maintain healthy sun habits. The advice in this book isn't so strange, is it? Try and see for yourself if it doesn't make you healthier and thinner than you had anticipated. Please visit Dietdoctor.com and tell me how it goes.

Good luck!

Acknowledgments

To Garry Taubes, whose book *Good Calories, Bad Calories* made me irrevocably swallow the red pill. This book would not have happened without it.

Michael Pollan for the vaccination against reversed nutritonism and the focus on real food.

The giants whose shoulders we stand upon: William Banting, Weston A. Price, Thomas Latimer Cleave, John Yudkin, and Robert Atkins (to name a few). The title of the book can be considered an homage to *Dr. Atkins' Diet Revolution* from 1972, the year I was born.

Kerstin Bergfors, my publisher, for all the encouragement and because you are never prematurely satisfied. Cecilia Hellberg, my editor, for hundreds of irritating objections that resulted in a much better book.

Dr. Eric Westman and Dr. Michael D. Fox for incredible hospitality, even by American standards.

My blog readers for 332 comments with suggestions when I asked them for book title suggestions. They had many good suggestions, and many were similar to the final title. The first person to suggest *The High-Fat, Low-Carb Food Revolution* was Diana Olofsson, so a special thank you goes to her.

Ulla Holmgren, who came up with the name the Diet Doctor. A big thank you!

A special thanks for Nicklas @ näringslara, Mikael Jansson, Kenneth Ekdahl, hemul, JAUS, patrik, Lund, Erik Kilborn, Kattmoster, and many others for discussions and advice. Thanks to Trance, Viktor, Jabob Gudiol, and many others for objections that have forced me to refine my arguments, and the professors Claude Marcus, Stephan Rössner, and Mai-Lis Hellénius for past debates, for the same reasons.

For productive discussions about the topic of this book, in no particular order: Fredrik Nyström, Jonas Colting, William Davis, Mary Vernon, Jimmy Moore, Tom Naughton, Annika Dahlqvist, Lars-Erik Litsfeldt, Sten Sture Skaldeman, Karl Arfors, Ralf Sundberg, Uffe Ravnskov, Monique Forslund, Anna Hallén, Jonas Bergqvist, Christer Enkvist, Jan Hammarsten, Johan Frostegård, Fredrik Paulún, Bo Zackrisson, Per Wikholm, Anna J.D. Jacobsson, Margareta Lundström, Åsa Lundberg, Mats Forsenberg, Daniel Strandroth, Mats Wiman, Peter M. Nilsson, Jörgen Vesti Nielsen, Bitten Jonsson, Göran Adlén, Kennet Jacobsson, Lars Block, Jakob Skov, and Magnus Ehrsson.

Muse for the soundtrack during my writing.

Marie Eenfeldt for author inspiration, Erik Eenfeldt for a couple of hundred overnight stays in Stockholm, and Johan Eenfeldt for invaluable IT support.

And finally, thanks to Kristin. Neither I nor this book would have been the same without you.

Do you want to know more?

The Internet hosts vast amounts of free information. A good place to start is my blog, the world's biggest low-carb website, Dietdoctor.com.

Books

There are lots of good books. For those who really want to read up on the history and research of low-carbohydrate diets, I recommend Taubes's book.

Good Calories, Bad Calories by Gary Taubes. It is a thick book in English, but no one has written more extensively on the subject.

The Obesity Code by Dr. Jason Fung. Dr. Fung is a world-leading expert on intermittent fasting and LCHF. Weight gain and obesity are driven by hormones and only by understanding the effects of insulin and insulin resistance can we achieve lasting weight loss.

Lose Weight by Eating! by Sten Sture Skalderman. It contains advice about a strict low-carbohydrate diet.

General books about real food

In Defense of Food by Michael Pollan. A brilliant book about real food. I highly recommend it.

For great low-carb recipes, see dietdoctor.com/low-carb/recipes

References

The easiest way of finding and reading the reference is to go to www.dietdoctor.com. It has many direct links to the sources. To read the scientific studies that I refer to, you can also check out "PubMed" and search for them there.

Introduction

BERGLUND QUOTE
Fet mat orsakar inte övervikt, dn 091224. Se även: Berglund G, m.fl. *Fett och kardiovaskulär hälsa – är vi helt felinformerade?* Läkartidningen. 2007;104(49–50):3780–4.

I. In Retrospect

1. What are you designed to eat?

THE STORY OF ALBERT SCHWEITZER
Taubes G. *Good calories, Bad calories.* First Anchor Books edition 2008, p.89 ff.

LOREN CORDAIN'S ESTIMATES
Cordain L, et al. *Plant-animal subsistence ratios and macronutrient energy estimations in worldwide hunter-gatherer diets.* Am J Clin Nutr 2000;71:682–92.

REAL FOOD
Pollan M. *Till matens försvar. (In Defense of Food)* Ordfront förlag, 2009.

INSULIN LEVELS WITH OR WITHOUT NEW FOOD
Lindeberg S, et al. *Low serum insulin in traditional Pacific Islanders – the Kitava Study.* Metabolism. 1999 Oct;48(10):1216–9.

THE SUGAR CURVE

Data from Johnson RJ, et al. *Potential role of sugar (fructose) in the epidemic of hypertension, obesity and the metabolic syndrome, diabetes, kidney disease, and cardiovascular disease.* Am J Clin Nutr 2007;86:899–906.

NO CAVITIES DURING THE STONE AGE

For example, see Petra Mojnar's dissertation *Tracing Prehistoric Activities: Life ways, habitual behaviour and health of hunter-gatherers on Gotland,* Stockholm university 2008.

DANISCO SUGAR AND TEETH BRUSHING:

http://www.Dietdoctor.com/nyhetsockerarbra.

THE STORY OF T. L. CLEAVE

Taubes G. *Good calories, Bad calories.* First Anchor Books edition, 2008, p.112 ff.

2. The mistake, the fear of fat, and the obesity epidemic

1984

Taubes G. *Nutrition. The soft science of dietary fat.* Science. 2001 Mar 30;291(5513):2536–45.

ANCEL KEYS:

Meet Monsieur Cholesterol, Intervju ur Minnesota Update 1979. http://www.mbbnet.umn.edu/hoff/hoff_ak.html

SIX COUNTRIES

Keys A. *Atherosclerosis: A problem in newer public health.* J Mount Sinai Hosp 1953;20:118–39.

CALLING KEYS' BLUFF

Yerushalmy J, et al. *Fat in the diet and mortality from heart disease; a methodologic note.* NY State J Med. 1957 Jul 15;57(14):2343–54.

FOLLOWING UP ON SEVEN COUNTRIES

Keys A, et al. *The diet and 15-year death rate in the Seven Countries study.* Am J Epidemiol. 1986;124:903–15.

MUNICIPAL TAXES AND HEART DISEASE

Ravnskov R. *Fat and Cholesterol are Healthy.* Optimal förlag 2008, p. 29.

BEARDS AND HEART ATTACKS

Ebrahim S. et al. *Shaving, coronary heart disease, and stroke: the Caerphilly Study.* Am J Epidemiol. 2003 Feb 1;157(3):234–8.

YUDKIN'S STORY

Taubes G. *Good calories, Bad calories.* First Anchor Books edition, 2008, p. 119 ff.

KEYS' EXECUTION OF YUDKIN

Keys A. *Sucrose in the diet and coronary heart disease.* Atherosclerosis 1971; 14:193–202. referenser 237

BURKITT AND FIBER

Burkitt DP, et al. *Effect of dietary fibre on stools and the transit-times, and its role in the causation of disease.* Lancet. 1972 Dec 30;2(7792):1408–12.

Story JA, et al. Denis Parsons Burkitt (1911–1993). J Nutr. 1994 Sep;124(9):1551–4.

POLITICIANS DECIDE THINGS, THE HUNT FOR EVIDENCE, ETC.
Taubes G. Nutrition. *The soft science of dietary fat.*
Science. 2001 Mar 30;291(5513):2536–45.

Taubes G. "What if It's All Been a Big Fat Lie?", *New York Times* 020707: http://www.
nytimes.com/2002/07/07/magazine/whatifitsallbeenabigfatlie.html

THE AMERICAN OBESITY EPIDEMIC
Wang Y, et al. *Will All Americans Become Overweight or Obese? Estimating the
Progression and Cost of the us Obesity Epidemic.* Obesity (2008) 16 10, 2323–2330.

THE SWEDISH OBESITY EPIDEMIC
SCB:s ulfundersökningar1980–2002: http://www.scb.se/Pages/TableAndChar_4953l.aspx

Folkhälsoinstitutets folkhälsoenkät 2004–2009: http://www.fhi.se/
Statistikuppföljning/Nationellafolkhalsoenkaten/Levnadsvanor/overviktochfetma/

SWEDISH BUTTER SALES
Svensk mjölks statistik: http://www.svenskmjolk.se/Statistik/Mejeriochkonsumtion/
Smorochovrigtmatfett/

3. The demise of the world as we know it

QUOTE BY FREDRIK NYSTRÖM
Corren interview, September 2009. Also see his book *Ät upp till bevis.*
Optimal förlag, 2010.

THE WHI STUDY:
Howard BV, et al. *Low-Fat Dietary Pattern and Risk of Cardiovascular Disease.
The Women's Health Initiative Randomized Controlled Dietary Modification Trial.*
JAMA. 2006;295.655–666.

QUOTE BY KARIN BOJS:
Low Fat does not reduce the risk of disease, DN 060207.

INCREASED RISK FOR THE HEART DISEASED
P. 661, the first paragraph of the WHI study. As commented in:
Mozaffarian D. *Low-Fat Diet and Cardiovascular Disease.* JAMA. 2006;296(3):279.

THE CONTENTS OF BREAST MILK
http://www.fineli.fi/food.php?foodid=603&lang=sv

MORE ADDITIVES IN KEYHOLE PRODUCTS
http://www.svd.se/nyheter/vetenskap/matklimat/vad-sager-markningen-om-
tillsatser_3398997.svd

THE CONTEST FOR THE MOST E-SUBSTANCES
http://hakkesnack.blogsome.com/2008/05/01/tavlingsresultat-flest-e-nummer

KEYHOLE PRODUCTS "LOW FAT YOGURT" FILLED WITH SUGAR
P. 3 in the Swedish FDAcharter LIVSFS 2009:6.

THE NATIONAL CHEF TEAM AND MARGARINE
http://www.Dietdoctor.com/kocklandslagetdumparmargarinet

http://www.svd.se/naringsliv/nyheter/konsten-att-inte-lyckas-samarbeta_3470059.svd

SCRUTINIZING THE 72/8 LIST
NFA should stop with dietary advice to the public, Dagens Medicin 090408.
http://www.dagensmedicin.se/asikter/debatt/2009/04/08/livsmedelsverket-bor-omede/index.xml

SLV "AVOIDS RESPONSIBILITY"
From the 090909: http://www.dagensmedicin.se/asikter/ledare2/2009/09/09/kvinnliga-lakarloner-en-sk/index.xml

PROMISE AND THE HEART AND LUNG FUND
http://www.Dietdoctor.com/hjar-tlungfonden-dumpar-becel

QUOTE BY ROGER HÖGLUND
From Dagens Medicin 090213. http://www.dagensmedicin.se/nyheter/2009/02/13/hjart-lungfonden-bryter-me/index.xml

THE FIRST REVIEW
Mente, et al. *A Systematic Review of the Evidence Supporting a Causal Link Between Dietary Factors and Coronary Heart Disease.* Arch Intern Med. 2009;169(7):659–669.

THE WHO REPORT
Skeaff CM, et al. *Dietary Fat and Coronary Heart Disease: Summary of Evidence from Prospective Cohort and Randomised Controlled Trials.* Ann Nutr Metab 2009;55:173–201.

THE THIRD REVIEW
SiriTarino PW, et al. *Meta-analysis of prospective cohort studies evaluating the association of saturated fat with cardiovascular disease.* Am J Clin Nutr. 2010 Jan 13. [Epub ahead of print]

QUOTE BY PETER M. NILSSON
http://www.Dietdoctor.com/annuenprofessordagsattsattapunkt

QUOTE BY JOHAN FROSTEGÅRD
Lose weight with the Professor's method, Expressen 100111.

II. Forward

4. A new but old solution

WILLIAM BANTING
Banting's *Letter on corpulence* can be found online.

QUOTE BY MARTIN INGVAR:
Ingvar M. *Watch your weight,* Natur & Kultur, 2010, p. 73.

ATKINS
http://www.nytimes.com/2003/04/18/nyregion/dr-robert-c-atkins-author-controversial-but-best-selling-diet-books-dead-72.html

STRANGE DEBATE ARTICLE
Marcus C, et al. *Kost med högt intag av fett kan ifrågasättas.* Läkartidningen. 2008; 105(24–25):1864–6.

CONTINUED DEBATE:
Eenfeldt A. *Märkligt utspel från kostexperter.* Läkartidningen 2008; 105(30–31); 2118–20.

Marcus C, et al. *Ett inlägg ägnat att förvirra.* Läkartidningen 2008;105(30-31);2119–20.

Eenfeldt A. *Hög tid för nytänkande i kostfrågan.* Läkartidningen 2008 Sep 10–16;105(37):2496–7.

Marcus C, et al. *Oroande att extremkost marknadsförs i sjukvården.* 2008 Sep 17-23;105(38):2590-1.

Sundberg R, et al. *Lågkolhydratkost vid diabetes och fetma är en fysiologisk och evidensbaserad metod.* Läkartidningen 2008 Nov 19–25;105(47):3460–1.

BAD LONG TERM EFFECTS FROM COUNTING CALORIES:
SBU. *Fetma – problem och åtgärder.* 2002

5. Weight loss without hunger

CHRISTER ENKVIST
Fel att vi blir feta av fett, dn Debatt 2004:
http://www.birkastaff.eu/doc/doc_old/html/a_fetEnkvist.htm

DIETING GEL
Food scientists develop appetite-curbing gel. The Guardian 100119. http://www.guardian.co.uk/education/2010/jan/19/gel-curb-appetite-scientists

OBESITY EPIDEMIC AMONG BABIES
Kim J, et al. *Trends in Overweight from 1980 through 2001 among Preschool-Aged Children Enrolled in a Health Maintenance Organization.* Obesity (Silver Spring). 2006 Jul;14(7):1107–12.

GÖRAN ADLÉN
www.Dietdoctor.com/?s=adlén

PETS, CARNIVORES, BEARS, AND PIGS
Mer i intervju med doktor Christer Enkvist: www.Dietdoctor.com/om-smala-grisar-och-feta-manniskor

AMERICA AND ISRAEL
Gardner CD, et al. *Comparison of the Atkins, Zone, Ornish, and learn Diets for Change in Weight and Related Risk Factors Among Overweight Premenopausal Women.* The a to z Weight Loss Study: A Randomized Trial. JAMA. 2007;297:969–977.

Shai I, et al. *Weight loss with a low-carbohydrate, mediterranean, or low-fat diet.* N Engl J Med 2008;359(3);229–41.

TWENTY ONE RANDOMIZED STUDIES AND TWO META ANALYSES
Sondike SB, et al. *Effects of a low-carbohydrate diet on weight loss and cardiovascular risk factor in overweight adolescents.* J Pediatr. 2003 Mar;142(3):253–8.

Brehm BJ, et al. *A Randomized Trial Comparing a Very Low Carbohydrate Diet and a Calorie-Restricted Low Fat Diet on Body Weight and Cardiovascular Risk Factors in Healthy Women.* J Clin Endocrinol Metab 2003; 88:1617–1623.

Foster GD, et al. *A Randomized Trial of a Low-Carbohydrate Diet for Obesity.* N Engl J Med 2003; 348:2082-90.

Samaha FF, et al. *A Low-Carbohydrate as Compared with a Low-Fat Diet in Severe Obesity.* N Engl J Med 2003; 348:2074–81.

Sondike SB, et al. *Effects of a low-carbohydrate diet on weight loss and cardiovascular risk factor in overweight adolescents.* J Pediatr. 2003 Mar; 142(3):253–8.

Aude YW, et al. *The National Cholesterol Education Program Diet vs a Diet Lower in Carbohydrates and Higher in Protein and Monounsaturated Fat. A Randomized Trial.* Arch Intern Med. 2004;164:2141–2146.

Volek JS, et al. *Comparison of energy-restricted very low-carbohydrate and low-fat diets on weight loss and body composition in overweight men and women.* Nutrition & Metabolism 2004, 1:13.

Meckling KA, et al. *Comparison of a Low-Fat Diet to a Low-Carbohydrate Diet on Weight Loss, Body Composition, and Risk Factors for Diabetes and Cardiovascular Disease in Free-Living, Overweight Men and Women.* J Clin Endocrinol Metab 2004;89: 2717–2723.

Yancy WS Jr, et al. *A Low-Carbohydrate, Ketogenic Diet versus a Low-Fat Diet To Treat Obesity and Hyperlipidemia. A Randomized, Controlled Trial.* Ann Intern Med. 2004;140:769–777.

Stern L, et al. *The Effects of Low-Carbohydrate versus Conventional Weight Loss Diets in Severely Obese Adults: One-Year Follow-up of a Randomized Trial.* Ann Intern Med. 2004;140:778–785.

Nichols-Richardsson SM, et al. *Perceived Hunger Is Lower and Weight Loss Is Greater in Overweight Premenopausal Women Consuming a Low-Carbohydrate/High-Protein vs High-Carbohydrate/Low-Fat Diet.* J Am Diet Assoc. 2005;105:1433–1437.

Dansinger ML, et al. *Comparison of the Atkins, Ornish, Weight Watchers, and Zone Diets for Weight Loss and Heart Disease Risk Reduction. A Randomized Trial.* JAMA. 2005;293:43–53.

Truby H, et al. *Randomised controlled trial of four commercial weight loss programmes in the uk: initial findings from the bbc "diet trials".* bmj. 2006 Jun 3;332(7553):1309–14.

Gardner CD, et al. *Comparison of the Atkins, Zone, Ornish, and learn Diets for Change in Weight and Related Risk Factors Among Overweight Premenopausal Women. The a to z Weight Loss Study: A Randomized Trial.* JAMA. 2007;297:969–977.

Ebbeling CB, et al. *Effects of a Low–Glycemic Load vs Low-Fat Diet in Obese Young Adults. A Randomized Trial.* JAMA. 2007; 297:2092-2102.

Shai I, et al. *Weight loss with a low-carbohydrate, mediterranean, or low-fat diet.* N Engl J Med 2008; 359(3);229–41.

Sacks FM, et al. *Comparison of Weight-Loss Diets with Different Compositions of Fat, Protein, and Carbohydrates.* N Engl J Med 2009; 360:859–73.

Brinkworth GD, et al. *Long-term effects of a very-low-carbohydrate weight loss diet compared with an isocaloric low-fat diet after 12 mo.* Am J Clin Nutr 2009;90:23–32.

Frisch S, et al. *A randomized controlled trial on the efficacy of carbohydrate-reduced or fat-reduced diets in patients attending a telemedically guided weight loss program.* Cardiovascular Diabetology 2009, 8:36.

Yancy WS Jr, et al. *A Randomized Trial of a Low-Carbohydrate Diet vs Orlistat Plus a Low-Fat Diet for Weight Loss.* Arch Intern Med. 2010;170(2):136–145.

Foster GD, et al. *Weight and Metabolic Outcomes After 2 Years on a Low-Carbohydrate Versus Low-Fat Diet. A Randomized Trial.* Ann Intern Med. 2010; 153:147–157.

Krebs NF, et al. *Efficacy and Safety of a High Protein, Low Carbohydrate Diet for Weight Loss in Severely Obese Adolescents.* J Pediatr 2010; 157:252-8.

Nordmann AJ, et al. *Effects of Low-Carbohydrate vs Low-Fat Diets on Weight Loss and Cardiovascular Risk Factors. A Meta-analysis of Randomized Controlled Trials.* Arch Intern Med. 2006; 166:285–293.

Hession M, et al. *Systematic review of randomized controlled trials of low-carbohydrate vs. low-fat/low-calorie diets in the management of obesity and its comorbidities.* Obes Rev. 2009 Jan; 10(1):36–50. Epub 2008 Aug 11.

THE WOMEN IN THE SACHS STUDY
Bilder: http://www.Dietdoctor.com/okand-dynamit-till-kostdebatten

QUOTE BY MARIN INGVAR
Ingvar M. *Hjärnkoll på vikten,* Natur & Kultur, 2010, p.72.

SOLVEIG'S STORY
Hexeberg, S. *Ekstrem vektreduksjon uten kirurgi.* Tidsskr Nor Laegeforen. 2009 Dec 3; 129(23):2497.

THE STORY OF JONAS TAGG
Jonas gick ner 92 kilo med fettdiet, Expressen 090322.

THE STORY OF DANIEL STRANDROTH
http://www.Dietdoctor.com/hur-man-gar-ner-50-kil

THE KUWAIT STORY
Dashti HM, et al. *Long term effects of ketogenic diet in obese subjects with high cholesterol level.* Mol Cell Biochem. 2006 Jun; 286(1–2):1–9.

SPANISH KETOGENIC MEDITERRANEAN DIET
PérezGuisado J, et al. *Spanish Ketogenic Mediterranean Diet: a healthy cardiovascular diet for weight loss.* Nutr J. 2008 Oct 26; 7:30.

THE RELATIVELY SMALL EFFECT OF EXERCISE ON WEIGHT
Simple summary in Time Magazine 090809, *Why Exercise Won't Make You Thin*; http://www.time.com/time/health/article/0,8599,1914857,00.html

USELESS TO GIVE ADVICE TO »FAT PEOPLE«
www.Dietdoctor.com/ingen-ide-ge-rad-till-fetknoppar

CANDY IN PHARMACIES
Apoteket lurar feta att äta godis, Västerås läns tidning 091029.

QUOTE BY STEPHAN RÖSSNER, »SQUARE ONE ONCE AGAIN«
Mörk framtid för fetmapiller, svd 100409. http://www.svd.se/nyheter/inrikes/mork-framtid-for-fetmapiller_4540501.svd

VITAMIN B DEFICIENCY AFTER GBP
Schroeder M, et al. *Tidig komplikation efter överviktskirurgi. Wernickes encefalopati uppstod inom tre månader hos 23-årig kvinna.* Läkartidningen. 2009 Sep 2–8;106(36):2216–7.

Aasheim ET. *Wernicke encephalopathy after bariatric surgery – a systematic review.*

Ann Surg. 2008;248:714–20.

OTHER DEFICIENCIES AFTER GBP
Matrana MR, et al. *Vitamin deficiency after gastric bypass surgery: a review.* South Med J. 2009 Oct; 102(10):1025–31.

OSTEOPOROSIS AFTER GBP
Wang A, et al. *The effects of obesity surgery on bone metabolism: what orthopedic surgeons need to know.* Am J Orthop. 2009 Feb;38(2):77–9.

BRAIN SURGERY FOR OBESITY
http://www.Dietdoctor.com/hjarnkirurgi-nya-behandlingen-mot-fetma

6. Diabetes and an end to the madness

QUOTE BY FREDRIK NYSTRÖM
Interview in Dagens Medicin nr 10, 2009.

KENNET JACOBSSON
Läs mer på www.Dietdoctor.com/ett-samtal-vid-mejeridisken respektively www.kennetjacobsson.se

A HEALTH DISASTER
The number of diabetes, as estimated by the WHO in 1985,95: http://www.who.int/diet-physicalactivity/publications/facts/diabetes/en/2010 and 2030 from IDF *Diabetes Atlas* 4th ed. International Diabetes Federation, 2009.

Quote by Mbayana from pressrelease IDF October 2009: http://www.idf.org/latest-diabe-tes-figures-paint-grim-global-picture

"CUCUMBER AND LARD"
The SBU report "Mat vid diabetes" May 2010, p. 31.

THE PETRÉN DIET AND AN EXTRA SIDE OF PORK
Östman J. *Från svältkurer till pankreastransplantationer. Diabetesbehandlingen i ett 100-årigt perspektiv.* Läkartidningen 2004; 101:4229–3, 4233–7.

"DIABETIC COOKERY", COOKBOOK FROM 1917
Can be read for free at http://www.archive.org/details/diabeticcookeryrooooppeiala

"EVIDENCE BASED" EUROPEAN DIETARY ADVICE
Mann JI, et al. *Evidence-based nutritional approaches to the treatment and prevention of diabetes mellitus.* Nutr Metab Cardiovasc Dis. 2004; 14:373–94.

"No scientific evidence" according to SBU: the SBU report *Mat vid diabetes*, May 2010, summary and conclusions.

LOWER BLOOD SUGAR AND FEWER CARBOHYDRATES
Boden G, et al. *Effect of a Low-Carbohydrate Diet on Appetite, Blood Glucose Levels, and Insulin Resistance in Obese Patients with Type 2 Diabetes.* Ann Intern Med. 2005;142:403–411.

Hertzler SR, et al. *Glycemic and insulinemic response to energy bars of differing macronutrient composition in healthy adults.* Medical Science Monitor 2003;9:cr84–90.

Noakes M, et al. *Comparison of isocaloric very low carbohydrate/high saturated fat and high carbohydrate/low saturated fat diets on body composition and cardiovascular risk.* Nutr Metab (Lond). 2006 Jan 11;3:7.

INTENSIVE TREATMENT THAT KILLS DIABETICS
Accord Study Group, et al. *Effect of intensive glucose lowering in type 2 diabetes.*
N Engl J Med. 2008 Jun 12; 358(24):2545–59.

THE STORY OF JÖRGEN VESTI NIELSENS
Litsfeldt, LE. *Fettskrämd*, 3:e upplagan, Optimal förlag, 2007, chapter 9.

THE KARLSHAMN STUDY
Nielsen JV, et al. *Low-carbohydrate diet in type 2 diabetes: stable improvement of
bodyweight and glycemic control during 44 months follow-up.* Nutr Metab (Lond).
2008 May 22; 5:14.

NINE RANDOMIZED STUDIES ON CARBOHYDRATE INTAKE OF TYPE 2 DIABETICS
Stern L, et al. *The effects of low-carbohydrate versus conventional weight loss diets in
severely obese adults: one-year follow-up of a randomized trial.* Ann Intern Med
2004; 140:778–85.

Daly ME, et al. *Short-term effects of severe dietary carbohydrate-restriction advice in
Type 2 diabetes–a randomized controlled trial.* Diabet Med. 2006 Jan;23(1):15–20.

Wolever TM, et al. *The Canadian Trial of Carbohydrates in Diabetes (ccd), a 1-y
controlled trial of lowglycemic-index dietary carbohydrate in type 2 diabetes: no
effect on glycated hemoglobin but reduction in c-reactive protein.* Am J Clin Nutr
2008; 87:114–25.

Shai I, et al. *Weight Loss with a Low-Carbohydrate, Mediterranean, or Low-Fat Diet.*
N Engl J Med. 2008 Jul 17; 359(3):229–41.

Westman EC, et al. *The effect of a low-carbohydrate, ketogenic diet versus a lowglycemic
index diet on glycemic control in type 2 diabetes mellitus.* Nutr. Metab
(Lond.) 2008 Dec 19; 5:36.

Jönsson T, et al. *Beneficial effects of a Paleolithic diet on cardiovascular risk factors in
type 2 diabetes: a randomized cross-over pilot study.* Cardiovasc Diabetol. 2009 Jul
16;8:35.

Davis NJ, et al. *Comparative Study of the Effects of a 1-Year Dietary Intervention of a
Low-Carbohydrate Diet Versus a Low-Fat Diet on Weight and Glycemic Control in
Type 2 Diabetes.* Diabetes Care. 2009 Jul;32(7):1147–52.

Esposito K, et al. *Effects of a Mediterranean-Style Diet on the Need for Antihyperglycemic Drug
Therapy in Patients With Newly Diagnosed Type 2 Diabetes.* Ann Intern
Med. 2009 Sep 1;151(5):306–14.

Elhayanu A, et al. *A low carbohydrate Mediterranean diet improves cardiovascular risk factors
and diabetes control among overweight patients with type 2 diabetes mellitus: a 1-year
prospective randomized intervention study.* Diabetes Obes Metab.
2010 Mar; 12(3):204–9.

INTERVIEW WITH DR. WESTMAN
http://www.Dietdoctor.com/atkins-i-praktiken

THE IRONIC DEFENSE OF SBU
Korttidsstudier är vanskliga som grund till kostråd. Dagens Medicin debatt 100702: http://
www.dagensmedicin.se/asikter/debatt/2010/07/02/
sbuharpatienternashalsa/index.xml

MORE ABOUT THE SBU REVIEW

http://www.Dietdoctor.com/sbu-valj-mat-sjalv
http://www.Dietdoctor.com/inget-vetenskapligt-stod

NORMALIZE BLOOD SUGAR BEFORE WEIGHT LOSS

Boden G, et al. *Effect of a Low-Carbohydrate Diet on Appetite, Blood Glucose Levels, and Insulin Resistance in Obese Patients with Type 2 Diabetes.* Ann Intern Med. 2005;142:403–411.

LOW CARBOHYDRATE DIETS AND TYPE 1 DIABETES

Nielsen JV, et al. *A Low Carbohydrate Diet in Type 1 Diabetes: Clinical Experience – A Brief Report.* Uppsala J Med Sci 110 (3): 267–273, 2005.

THE BROCHURE "FOOD FOR DIABETICS"

Published by the Bayer Health Care Diabetes Care, revised in 2009.

7. The Western Diseases

THE STORY OF VILHJALMUR STEFANSSON

Adventures in diet, Harper's Monthly magazine, november 1935. Can be read online. Google it.

THE STORY OF JAY WORTMAN

http://www.drjaywortman.com/

THE DOCUMENTARY

My Big, Fat Diet (2008) Mystique films.
    Can be ordered at http://www.mystiquefilms.com/mbfd/

RESULTS FROM THE STUDY

http://www.cbc.ca/thelens/bigfatdiet/Poster.pdf

THE INTERHEART STUDY

Yusuf S, et al. *Effect of potentially modifiable risk factors associated with myocardial infarction in 52 countries (the interheart study): case-control study.* Lancet 2004; 364: 937–52.

THE DEFINITION OF METABOLIC SYNDROME

There are several different definitions of metabolic syndrome and they only vary in details. This one derives from NCEP ATP-III.

THE PREVALENCE OF METABOLIC SYNDROME IN USA

Ervin RB. *Prevalence of metabolic syndrome among adults 20 years of age and over, by sex, age, race and ethnicity, and body mass index: United States, 2003–2006.* Natl Health Stat Report. 2009 May 5; (13):1–7.

THE MEDICATION OF ELDERLY SWEDES

Folkhälsoinstitutet. Nationella folkhälsoenkäten 2008. http://www.fhi.se/Documents/ Statistik-uppfoljning/Folkhalsoenkaten/Resultat-2008/Lakemedelsanvandning.pdf

A PERFECT CORRELATION, STUDIES

The same studies as in chapter five so please refer to those citations.

THE WHI STUDY

See the citations in chapter 3.

THE HARVARD STUDY

Mozzafarian D, et al. *Dietary fats, carbohydrate, and progression of coronary atherosclerosis in postmenopausal women.* Am J Clin Nutr 2004; 80:1175–84.

NURSE'S HEALTH STUDIES

Halton TL, et al. *Low-Carbohydrate-Diet Score and the Risk of Coronary Heart*

Disease in Women. N Engl J Med 2006; 355:1991–2002.

ULTRASONIC EXAMINATION OF BLOOD VESSELS
Shai I, et al. *Dietary Intervention to Reverse Carotid Atherosclerosis.* Circulation. 2010; 121:1200–1208.

THE STORY OF CHARLIE ABRAHAMS
www.charliefoundation.org

STUDIES ON LOW CARBOHYDRATE DIETS AND EPILEPSY
Kossoff EH, et al. *More fat and fewer seizures: dietary therapies for epilepsy.* Lancet Neurol. 2004 Jul; 3(7):415–20.

Kossoff EH, et al. *A prospective study of the modified Atkins diet for intractable epilepsy in adults.* Epilepsia 2008; 49(2):316–319.

SENSITIVE INTESTINES AND LOW CARBOHYDRATE DIETS
Austin GL, et al. *A Very Low-Carbohydrate Diet Improves Symptoms and Quality of Life in Diarrhea-Predominant Irritable Bowel Syndrome.* Clin Gastroenterol Hepatol. 2009 Jun;7(6):706–708.

HEARTBURN AND LOW CARBOHYDRATE DIETS
Austin GL, et al. *A very low-carbohydrate diet improves gastroesophageal reflux and its symptoms.* Dig Dis Sci. 2006 Aug; 51(8):1307–12.

PCOS AFFECT EVERY TENTH WOMAN
Teede H, et al. *Polycystic ovary syndrome: a complex condition with psychological, reproductive and metabolic manifestations that impacts on health across the lifespan.* bmc Med. 2010 Jun 30;8:41.

PCOS AND GI DIETS
Marsh KA, et al. *Effect of a low glycemic index compared with a conventional healthy diet on polycystic ovary syndrome.* Am J Clin Nutr. 2010 Jul;92(1):83–92.

PCOS AND LOW CARBOHYDRATE DIETS
Mavropoulos JC, et al. *The effects of a low-carbohydrate, ketogenic diet on the polycystic ovary syndrome: A pilot study.* Nutrition & Metabolism 2005, 2:35.

MALE PROBLEMS IN EVERY THIRD MAN
Stranne J, et al. *One-third of the Swedish male population over 50 years of age suffers from lower urinary tract symptoms.* Scand J Urol Nephrol. 2009;43(3):199–205.

LECTURE AND INTERVIEW WITH JAN HAMMARSTEN
http://www.Dietdoctor.com/maten-prostatan-och-halsan

HAMMARSTEN'S STUDY ABOUT PROSTATE DISEASES AND METABOLIC SYNDROME
Hammarsten J, et al. *Components of the metabolic syndrome-risk factors for the development of benign prostatic hyperplasia.* Prostate Cancer Prostatic Dis. 1998 Mar;1(3):157–162.

Hammarsten J, et al. *Clinical, haemodynamic, anthropometric, metabolic and insulin profile of men with high-stage and high-grade clinical prostate cancer.* Blood Press. 2004;13(1):47–55.

Hammarsten J, et al. *Hyperinsulinaemia: a prospective risk factor for lethal clinical prostate cancer.* Eur J Cancer. 2005 Dec; 41(18):2887–95.

Hammarsten J, et al. *Insulin and free oestradiol are independent risk factors for benign prostatic hyperplasia.* Prostate Cancer Prostatic Dis. 2009; 12(2):160–5.

Hammarsten J, et al. *A higher prediagnostic insulin level is a prospective risk factor for inci-*

dent prostate cancer. Cancer Epidemiol. 2010 Oct; 34(5):574–9.

CANCER AMONG NATIVE POPULATIONS
Taubes G. *Good calories, Bad calories,* First Anchor Books edition, September 2008, p. 89-95.

CANCER IN THE WHI STUDY
Pretice RL, et al. *Low-fat dietary pattern and risk of invasive breast cancer: the Women's Health Initiative Randomized Controlled Dietary Modification Trial.* JAMA. 2006 Feb 8; 295(6):629–42.

Beresford SA, et al. *Low-fat dietary pattern and risk of colorectal cancer: the Women's Health Initiative Randomized Controlled Dietary Modification Trial.* JAMA. 2006 Feb 8; 295(6):643–54.

LOW-FAT DIET FOR WOMEN WHO PREIVOUSLY SUFFERED FROM BREAST CANCER
Pierce JP, et al. *Influence of a Diet Very High in Vegetables, Fruit, and Fiber and Low in Fat on Prognosis Following Treatment for Breast Cancer. The Women's Healthy Eating and Living (WHEL) Randomized Trial.* JAMA. 2007; 298:289–298.

OBESE PEOPLE AND DIABETICS MORE OFTEN SUFFER FROM CANCER, THE CORRELATION WITH INSULIN/IGF
Giovannucci E, et al. *Diabetes and cancer: a consensus report.* Diabetes Care. 2010 Jul;33(7):1674–85.

LeRoith D, et al. *Obesity and type 2 diabetes are associated with an increased risk of developing cancer and a worse prognosis; epidemiological and mechanistic evidence. Exp Clin Endocrinol Diabetes.* 2008 Sep;116 Suppl 1:S4–6.

5 450 WOMEN ...
Kabat KC, et al. *Repeated measures of serum glucose and insulin in relation to postmenopausal breast cancer.* Int J Cancer. 2009 Jun 2. [Epub ahead of print]

STUDY FROM UMEÅ UNIVERSITY
Stocks T, et al. *Blood glucose and risk of incident and fatal cancer in the metabolic syndrome and cancer project (Me–Can): analysis of six prospective cohorts.* PLoS Med 2009 6(12): e1000201. doi:10.1371/journal.pmed.1000201

TWO REVIEWS IN AJCN
Gnagnarella P, et al. *Glycemic index, glycemic load, and cancer risk: a meta-analysis.* Am J Clin Nutr. 2008 Jun; 87(6):1793–801.

Barclay AW, et al. *Glycemic index, glycemic load, and chonic disease risk – a metaanalysis of observational studies.* Am J Clin Nutr. 2008 Mar; 87(3):627–37.

8. Cholesterol: killing the dragon

QUOTE BY RONALD KRAUSS
Your Unstoppable Heart, Men's Health 2010. http://www.menshealth.com/men/health/heart-disease/understanding-cholesterol-and-heart-disease/article/34cf5983f7a75210vg nvcm10000030281eac

SCRUTINIZING PROMISE'S MARKETING CAMPAIGN
Becel försökte mörklägga skillnader, Piteå Tidningen 081115.
http://www.piteatidningen.se/nyheter/artikel.aspx?ArticleId=4171670

Hundratals kan ha fått falska mätvärden, Piteå Tidningen 081116.
http://www.piteatidningen.se/nyheter/artikel.aspx?articleid=4171218

Läkare i norr varnar butiker för kolesterolkampanj, Dagens Medicin 081117.
http://www.dagensmedicin.se/nyheter/2008/11/17/butikerstallerinbecelk/index.xml

Becels turné stoppad efter pt:s avslöjande, Piteå Tidningen 081118.
http://www.piteatidningen.se/nyheter/artikel.aspx?articleid=4179241

THE MAJORITY OF ADULT SWEDES HAVE A CHOLESTEROL ABOVE 5
Wahlberg G. *Allmänläkarens dilemma: Det totala serumkolesterolvärdet mellan 5 och 8 mmol/l*. Läkartidningen. 2008 Oct 1–7; 105(40):2788–9.

PROMISE'S COMMERCIALS FOUND GUILTY
Böter i Danmark: Forbrugerrådet 081218 »Becelprodukter får bøde på 40 000 kroner«.
http://www.forbrugerraadet.dk/?cid=5764&ref=2820

The Advertising Ombudsman's verdicts: Case 0903-62 from 090917 and case 0902-05 from 090428.

The Market Ethics Councils verdict: statement 44/2008 – Dnr 04/2008.

THE PROPOSAL ABOUT »MCSTATIN«
Ferenczi EA, et al. *Can a Statin Neutralize the Cardiovascular Risk of Unhealthy Dietary Choices?* Am J Cardiol. 2010 Aug 15;106(4):587–592.

STATINS AND IMPOTENCE
Solomon H, et al. *Erectile dysfunction and statin treatment in high cardiovascular risk patients*. Int J Clin Pract. 2006 Feb; 60(2):141–5.

Do C, et al. *Statins and erectile dysfunction: results of a case/non-case study using the French Pharmacovigilance System Database*. Drug Saf. 2009;32(7):591–7.

STATINS AND MENTAL CLARITY:
Muldoon MF, et al. *Randomized trial of the effects of simvastatin on cognitive functioning in hypercholesterolemic adults*. Am J Med. 2004 Dec 1;117(11):823–9.

STATINS AND DIABETES
Sattar N, et al. *Statins and risk of incident diabetes: a collaborative meta-analysis of randomised statin trials*. Lancet. 2010 Feb 27; 375(9716):735–42.

INSULIN INCREASES HMGR
Ness GC, Chambers CM. *Feedback and hormonal regulation of hepatic 3-hydroxy-3-methylglutaryl coenzyme A reductase: the concept of cholesterol buffering capacity*. Proc Soc Exp Biol Med. 2000 May; 224(1):8–19.

THE STUDIES BEHIND THE NEW PERSPECTIVE ON CHOLESTEROL
A good summary that refers to the most important studies behind it:
Musunuru K. *Atherogenic Dyslipidemia: Cardiovascular Risk and Dietary Intervention*. Lipids (2010) 45:907–914.

THE DIVISION OF CHOLESTEROL (CHOLESTEROL/HDL ELLER APO RATIO) IS MORE IMPORTANT THAN THE CHOLESTEROL LEVEL OR LDL:
See Musunuru 2010 above in addition to: Lewington S, et al. *Blood cholesterol and vascular mortalityby age, sex, and blood pressure: a meta-analysis of individual data from 61 prospective studies with 55,000 vascular deaths*. Lancet. 2007 Dec 1; 370(9602):1829–39.

McQueen MJ, et al. *Lipids, lipoproteins, and apolipoproteins as risk markers of myocardial infarction in 52 countries (the interheart study): a case-control study*. Lancet. 2008 Jul 19;372(9634):224–33.

STATINS SIGNIFICANTLY REDUCE THE NUMBER OF DENSE LDL:
Bahadir MA, et al. *Effects of different statin treatments on small dense low-density lipoprotein in patients with metabolic syndrome.* J Atheroscler Thromb. 2009 Oct;16(5):684–90.

NO DEMONSTRATED BENEFIT FROM STATINS WITHOUT KNOWN HEART DISEASE
Kausik KR, et al. *Statins and All-Cause Mortality in High-Risk Primary Prevention. A Meta-analysis of 11 Randomized Controlled Trials Involving 65 229 Participants.* Arch Intern Med. 2010;170(12):1024–1031.

THE APO RATIO IS A SAFER MEASUREMENT OF RISK AS WELL AS THE DISTRIBUTION IN SWEDEN
Walldius G, et al. *Apolipoproteiner nya och bättre riskindikatorer för hjärtinfarkt.* Läkartidningen. 2004 Mar 25;101(13):1188–94.

BETTER APO RATIO WITH A LOW CARBOHYDRATE DIET
Shai I, et al. *Dietary Intervention to Reverse Carotid Atherosclerosis.* Circulation. 2010;121:1200–1208.

Jenkins D, et al. *The Effect of a Plant-Based Low-Carbohydrate (»Eco-Atkins«) Diet on Body Weight and Blood Lipid Concentrations in Hyperlipidemic Subjects.* Arch Intern Med. 2009;169(11):1046–1054.

9. A healthier future

CALMER STOMACHS FROM A LOW CARBOHYDRATE DIET
See the references in chapter 7

25 PROCENT OF CALORIES FROM JUNK FOOD
Livsmedelsverket. *Riksmaten – barn 2003. Livsmedels- och näringsintag bland barn i Sverige.* isbn: 91 7714 177 6.

A NUANCED VIEW FROM SKEPTICS
http://www.Dietdoctor.com/lchf-i-expressen-och-gt

THE STORY OF DR. THOMAS BOLTE
http://www.boltemedical.com/complementary_medicine_robert_atkins_md.htm

THE SCANDALOUS FOOD
Upphandlingen var olaglig, SvD 090702.
Sjukhusmaten är full av tillsatser, SvD 090511.
Sodexo putsade svar i matenkät, SvD 100916.

FAT IN BREASTMILK
Claims from the Finnish institute of health and wellfare's database available at www.fineli.fi

QUOTE FROM MARTIN INGVAR
Ingvar M. *Hjärnkoll på vikten.* Första upplagan, Natur och kultur, 2010, p. 86.

III. Guide

10. The Enjoyment Method/LCHF for beginners

MARGARINE, OMEGA 6, AND INFLAMMATORY DISEASES
See references in the section on questions and answers

11. Questions, answers, and myths

100 GRAM CARBOHYDRATES FOR THE BRAIN?
93 overweight people were randomly selected ...

Halyburton AK, et al. *Low- and high-carbohydrate weight-loss diets have similar effects on mood but not cognitive performance.* Am J Clin Nutr 2007; 86:580 –7.

106 OVERWEIGHT PEOPLE WERE RANDOMLY SELECTED ...
Brinkworth GD, et al. *Long-term Effects of a Very Low-Carbohydrate Diet and a Low-Fat Diet on Mood and Cognitive Function.* Arch Intern Med. 2009; 169(20):1873–1880.

EXERCISING ON A LOW CARBOHYDRATE DIET
Interview with Björn Ferry: http://www.Dietdoctor.com/att-ta-os-guld-pa-lagkolhydratkost

INTERVIEW WITH JIMMY LIDBERG
Brons för Jimmy Lidberg, dn 100906. http://www.dn.se/sport/brons-for-jimmy-lidberg1.1165826

ANTIOXIDANTS
ANALYSIS OF 67 STUDIES ...
Bjelakovic G, et al. *Antioxidant supplements for prevention of mortality in healthy participants and patients with various diseases.* Cochrane Database Syst Rev. 2008 Apr 16;(2):cd007176.

VITAMINS
The Swedish FDAs analysis of eggs: Press release Svenska ägg 090403: »Nya analyser från Livsmedelsverket visar: Påskägg – en riktig vitamininjektion«.

DOCUMENTED CASE OF SCURVY
Becker W. *Vitaminbrist mycket ovanligt i Sverige. d-vitamin till barn för att undvika rakit.* Läkartidningen 1997; 94: 2936–2940.

SWITCH TO POLYUNSATURATED FAT – TWO ANALYSES
Jacobsen MU, et al. *Major types of dietary fat and risk of coronary heart disease: a pooled analysis of 11 cohort studies.* Am J Clin Nutr 2009;89:1425–32.

Mozaffarian D, Micha R, Wallace S. *Effects on coronary heart disease of increasing polyunsaturated fat in place of saturated fat: a systematic review and meta-analysis of randomized controlled trials.* PLoS Med. 2010 Mar 23;7(3):e1000252.

MARGARINE, OMEGA 6, AND INFLAMMATORY DISEASES
Bolte G, et al. *Margarine consumption, asthma, and allergy in young adults: results of the German National Health Survey 1998.* Ann Epidemiol. 2005 Mar;15(3):207–13.

A STUDY CONDUCTED ON TWO-YEAR-OLD CHILDREN
Sausenthaler S, et al. *Margarine and butter consumption, eczema and allergic sensitization in children. The lisa birth cohort study.* Pediatr Allergy Immunol. 2006 Mar;17(2):85–93.

ULCEROUS COLITIS
Tjonneland A, et al. *Linoleic acid, a dietary n-6 polyunsaturated fatty acid, and the aetiology of ulcerative colitis: a nested case-control study within a European prospective cohort study.* Gut. 2009 Dec;58(12):1606–11. Epub 2009 Jul 23.

THREE MORE STUDIES:
Woods RK, et al. *Fatty acid levels and risk of asthma in young adults.* Thorax. 2004 Feb;59(2):105–10.

Bolte G, et al. *Margarine consumption and allergy in children.* Am J Respir Crit Care Med.

2001 Jan;163(1):277–9.

Trak-Fellermeier MA, et al. *Food and fatty acid intake and atopic disease in adults.* Eur Respir J. 2004 Apr;23(4):575–82.

THE UNILEVER YOUTUBE VIDEO:
http://www.youtube.com/watch?v=PkEigaUrx9U

THE FOOD OF SUMO WRESTLERS
Nishizawa T, et al. *Some factors related to obesity in the Japanese sumo wrestler.* Am J Clin Nutr 1976;29:1167–74.

PREGNANCY AND A LOW CARBOHYDRATE DIET
Hone J, et al. *Approach to the patient with Diabetes during Pregnancy.* J Clin Endocrinol Metab 2010 95:3578–85.

RENAL FUNCTIONALITY AND A LOW CARBOHYDRATE DIET
Brinkworth GD, et al. *Renal function following long-term weight loss in individuals with abdominal obesity on a very-low-carbohydrate diet vs high-carbohydrate diet.* J Am Diet Assoc. 2010 Apr; 110(4):633–8.

Vesti-Nielsen J, et al. *Lågkolhydratdiet hejdade njurfunktionsförsämring vid typ 2-diabetes.* Läkartidningen. 2008 Jul 23Aug 5; 105(30–31):2094–7.

OSTEOPOROSIS AND LOW CARBOHYDRATE DIETS
Carter JD, et al. *The effect of a low-carbohydrate diet on bone turnover.* Osteoporos Int. 2006;17(9):1398–403.

Foster GD, et al. *Weight and Metabolic Outcomes After 2 Years on a Low-Carbohydrate Versus Low-Fat Diet. A Randomized Trial.* Ann Intern Med. 2010;153:147–157.

Krebs NF, et al. *Efficacy and Safety of a High Protein, Low Carbohydrate Diet for Weight Loss in Severely Obese Adolescents.* J Pediatr 2010;157:252–8.

WHI AND CANCER
See the references in chapter seven.

RED MEAT AND CANCER
Alexander DD, et al. *Red meat and colorectal cancer: a critical summary of prospective epidemiologic studies.* Obes Rev. 2010 Jul 21. [Epub ahead of print]

12. *Advice for your weight*

DIET SODA AND EXCESS WEIGHT
Fowler SP, et al. *Fueling the Obesity Epidemic? Artificially Sweetened Beverage Use and Long-term Weight Gain.* Obesity (Silver Spring). 2008 Aug;16(8):1894–900.

STUDIES CONDUCTED ON RATS
Swithers SE, et al. *General and persistent effects of high-intensity sweeteners on body weight gain and caloric compensation in rats.* Behav Neurosci. 2009 August; 123(4): 772–780.

LOW CARBOHYDRATE DIETS AGAINST LOW FAT DIETS AND XENICAL
Yancy WS Jr, et al. *A randomized trial of a low-carbohydrate diet vs orlistat plus a lowfat diet for weight loss.* Arch Intern Med. 2010 Jan 25;170(2):136–45.

MULTIVITAMINS
Li Y, et al. *Effects of multivitamin and mineral supplementation on adiposity, energy expenditure and lipid profiles in obese Chinese women.* International Journal of Obesity (2010) 34, 1070–1077.

VITAMIN D AND INSULIN SENSITIVITY

von Hurst PR, et al. *Vitamin D supplementation reduces insulin resistance in South Asian women living in New Zealand who are insulin resistant and vitamin D deficient – a randomised, placebo-controlled trial.* British Journal of Nutrition (2010), 103:549–55.

FAT PEOPLE EAT MORE QUICKLY
Maruyama K, et al. *The joint impact on being overweight of self reported behaviours of eating quickly and eating until full: cross sectional survey.* BMJ 2008;337:a2002.

13. One last thing

VITAMIN D EXTENDS LIFE
Autier P, Gandini S. *Vitamin D supplementation and total mortality: a meta-analysis of randomized controlled trials.* Arch Intern Med. 2007 Sep 10;167(16):1730–7.

VITAMIN D PROTECTS AGAINS CANCER
Lappe JM, et al. *Vitamin d and calcium supplementation reduces cancer risk: results of a randomized trial.* Am J Clin Nutr. 2007 Jun; 85(6):1586–91.

VITAMIN D CAN HELP AGAINST DEPRESSION
Jorde R, et al. *Effects of vitamin D supplementation on symptoms of depression in overweight and obese subjects: randomized double blind trial.* J Intern Med. 2008 Dec; 264(6):599–609.

VITAMIN D AGAINST THE FLU
Urashima M, et al. *Randomized trial of vitamin d supplementation to prevent seasonal influenza a in schoolchildren.* Am J Clin Nutr. 2010 May; 91(5):1255–60.

VITAMIN D PREVENTS OSTEOPOROSIS
BischoffFerrari HA, et al. *Prevention of nonvertebral fractures with oral vitamin D and dose dependency: a meta-analysis of randomized controlled trials.* Arch Intern Med. 2009 Mar 23; 169(6):551–61.

VITAMIN D AND ATHLETE PERFORMANCE
Cannell JJ, et al. *Athletic performance and vitamin D.* Med Sci Sports Exerc. 2009 May; 41(5):1102–10.

www.Dietdoctor.com/mot-stanley-cup-seger-pa-d-vitamin

AUTISM AND THE DEBATE
Grant WB. *Epidemiologic evidence supporting the role of maternal vitamin d deficiency as a risk factor for the development of infantile autism.* Dermatoendocrinol. 2009 Jul;1(4):223–8.

Cannell JJ. *On the aetiology of autism.* Acta Paediatr. 2010 Aug; 99(8):1128–30.

Undvikandet av solljus har blivit en hälsorisk i DN Debatt 080715.

QUOTE BY OLA LARKÖ
Två glas solsken, tack!, Health Magazine 6, 2010.

VITAMIN D IS SAFE IN DOSES UP TO AT LEAST 10,000 E DAILY
Vieth, R. *Vitamin D supplementation, 25-hydroxyvitamin d concentrations, and safety.* Am J Clin Nutr 1999; 69:842–56.

Index